UNDERSTANDING INFECTIOUS DISEASES

Tracking the Causes and Spread of Infectious Diseases

Don Nardo

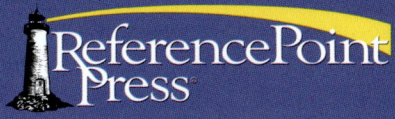

San Diego, CA

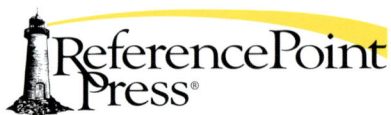

About the Author

Classical historian, amateur astronomer, and award-winning author Don Nardo has written numerous volumes about scientific topics, including *Destined for Space*, winner of the Eugene M. Emme Award for best astronomical literature; *Tycho Brahe*, winner of the National Science Teacher's Association's best book of the year; *Planet Under Siege*; *Climate Change*; *Deadliest Dinosaurs*; and *The History of Science*. Nardo, who also composes and arranges orchestral music, lives with his wife, Christine, in Massachusetts.

© 2022 ReferencePoint Press, Inc.
Printed in the United States

For more information, contact:
ReferencePoint Press, Inc.
PO Box 27779
San Diego, CA 92198
www.ReferencePointPress.com

ALL RIGHTS RESERVED.
No part of this work covered by the copyright hereon may be reproduced or used in any form or by any means—graphic, electronic, or mechanical, including photocopying, recording, taping, web distribution, or information storage retrieval systems—without the written permission of the publisher.

Picture Credits:
Cover: Kiselev Andrey Valerevich/Shutterstock.com

6: ©Look and Learn/Bridgeman Images
10: nullplus/iStock
14: Underwood Archives/UIG/Bridgeman Images
18: Tarker/Bridgeman Images
21: Anthony Bannister/NHPA/Photoshot/Newscom
25: Kateryna Kon/Shutterstock.com
27: Associated Press
32: Associated Press
34: CDC/Science Photo Library
38: ©SZ Photo/Waldemar Hauschild/Bridgeman Images
40: Malota/Shutterstock.com
44: Associated Press
46: Leonie Broekstra/Shutterstock.com
50: Jess Gregg/Shutterstock.com
53: faboi/Shutterstock.com

LIBRARY OF CONGRESS CATALOGING-IN-PUBLICATION DATA

Names: Nardo, Don, 1947- author.
Title: Tracking the causes and spread of infectious diseases / by Don Nardo.
Description: San Diego, CA : ReferencePoint Press, [2022] | Series: Understanding infectious diseases | Includes bibliographical references and index.
Identifiers: LCCN 2021008863 (print) | LCCN 2021008864 (ebook) | ISBN 9781678201647 (library binding) | ISBN 9781678201654 (ebook)
Subjects: LCSH: Epidemiology--Juvenile literature. | Communicable diseases--Epidemiology--Juvenile literature. | Epidemics--Juvenile literature. | Public health surveillance--Juvenile literature.
Classification: LCC RA653.5 .N37 2022 (print) | LCC RA653.5 (ebook) | DDC 614.4--dc23
LC record available at https://lccn.loc.gov/2021008863
LC ebook record available at https://lccn.loc.gov/2021008864

CONTENTS

Introduction   4
Birth of a New Medical Science

Chapter One   8
Disease Detectives' Basic Methods

Chapter Two   16
The Mystery of Sleeping Sickness

Chapter Three   23
The Mystery of Polio in the Blood

Chapter Four   30
The Mystery of the Dead Legionnaires

Chapter Five   36
The Mystery of HIV/AIDS

Chapter Six   42
The Mystery of Deadly Ebola in Africa

Chapter Seven   48
The Mystery of the Virus from Wuhan

Source Notes   55
Organizations and Websites   58
For Further Research   60
Index   62

INTRODUCTION

Birth of a New Medical Science

Before the mid-1800s, cholera—a disease that causes severe diarrhea and often death—was common in nearly every large European city. London, in southern England, was no exception. In 1853 close to eleven thousand people perished in scattered outbreaks of the disease in or near London. Individually, each of these epidemics paled in comparison to one that struck the city's Soho district beginning on August 31, 1854. A London physician who lived not far from Soho called it "the most terrible outbreak of cholera which ever occurred in the kingdom [of England.]"[1]

That doctor, John Snow, had recently gained some moderate fame, in part for helping the reigning monarch, Queen Victoria, through a difficult childbirth in 1853. Though generally well liked, Snow had sometimes been criticized by other medical experts. In particular, most of them felt that his ideas about cholera were misguided. The prevailing scientific explanation for that disease was that it was caused by miasma—a mass of corrupted, or tainted, air. Snow had suggested an alternative theory: that cholera derived from water that had somehow been contaminated.

A Trail of Clues

Thinking that the Soho outbreak might be a good place to test his theory, Snow took it upon himself to visit that neighborhood, a ten-minute walk from his own, mere days after the start of the outbreak. While he investigated, more and more people came down with cholera, and by September 7, 1854, the death toll from the ailment surpassed five hundred. Snow carefully searched for some sort of water source that might be causing the outbreak.

> **miasma**
>
> Refers to the idea of corrupted air or tainted air being the cause of cholera and several other diseases

The approach paid off. Snow initially noticed that nearly all the people who had come down with cholera lived within 250 yards (229 m) of the intersection of Cambridge Street and Broad Street. Moreover, in the midst of that intersection stood a public pump—an upright pipe bearing a handle. When someone pulled down on the handle, water from a well located below the pavement squirted up for the person to catch in a bucket.

Snow saw that this was where most neighborhood residents got their daily water for drinking, cooking, and bathing. He later recalled, "On proceeding to the spot, I found that nearly all the deaths had taken place within a short distance of the pump. There were only ten deaths in houses situated decidedly nearer to another street pump."[2]

As he continued to investigate, Snow uncovered a trail of other clues that seemed to support his theory. One consisted of his finding that two former residents of Soho, Susannah Eley and her niece, had also died in the outbreak. The two women had moved to another part of London years before. It made no sense to Snow, therefore, that they had perished from tainted air in Soho. Yet tellingly, both had liked the taste of the water from the Broad Street pump so much that they had daily sent a servant to fetch water from that source. This, Snow argued, was why they were the only residents of their own neighborhood to die of cholera during the Soho outbreak.

Further evidence for Snow's hypothesis came from examining the workers of the Lion Brewery, situated in the middle of Soho. None of the seventy employees got sick during the crisis. First, Snow said, if polluted air were behind the epidemic, why

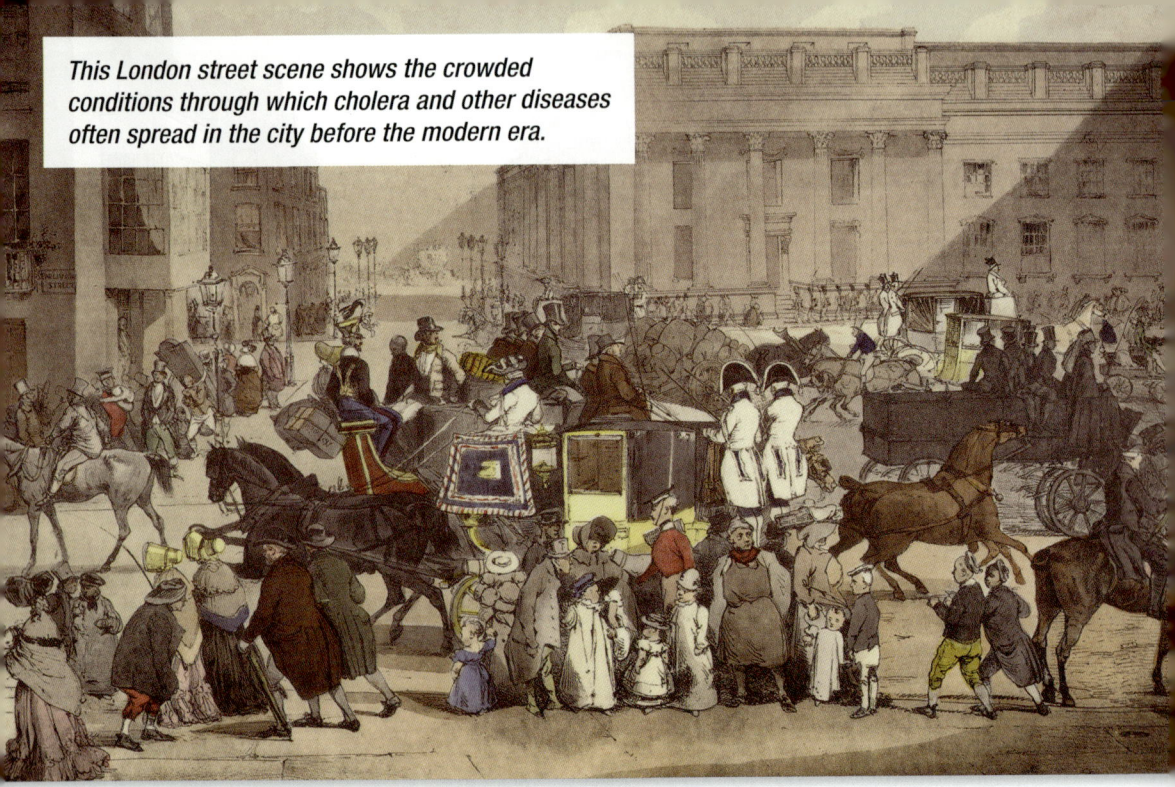

This London street scene shows the crowded conditions through which cholera and other diseases often spread in the city before the modern era.

had they been spared? Second, he went on, the brewery's owner regularly allowed his workers to drink free beer. What is more, the water used to make that brew came from the company's private well. Hence, those men never drank water from the Broad Street pump, which explained why they remained healthy during the outbreak.

Setting an Example for the Future

It turned out that Snow was right all along. Outbreaks of cholera in London and other English cities had indeed been caused by dangerous agents in local wells and other contaminated water sources. Snow did not know for sure what those agents were; nor did he ever find out, because he died in 1858. It was not until 1885, when scientists proved cholera is caused by a bacterium, that the full truth behind the Soho outbreak became known.

Nevertheless, Snow's hard work, cleverness, and dedication to the scientific method in a sense signaled the birth of a new medical science. Consisting of using various logical clues to track down the origins of diseases, it became known as epidemiology. Today epidemiologists, often called "disease detectives," have the benefit of advanced technologies of which Snow could never have dreamed. Yet his basic clue-gathering approach remains in use, and for that reason medical authorities around the globe remember him as the founder of epidemiology. One expert observer remarks that Snow's work "holds deep significance in today's society because his epidemiological research laid the foundation for controlling outbreaks of disease . . . [and his efforts] did an enormous amount of good for today's modern society."[3]

Snow himself had no idea that future generations would look back at him so fondly. But he did foresee that science would eventually uncover and understand the causes of disease, thereby saving untold millions of lives. "You and I may not live to see the day," he told a colleague, "but the time will arrive when great outbreaks of cholera will be things of the past; and it is the knowledge of the way in which the disease is propagated which will cause them to disappear."[4]

CHAPTER ONE

Disease Detectives' Basic Methods

When John Snow, the world's first true disease detective, was solving the mystery of what caused the 1854 cholera outbreak in London, scientists had known of the existence of germs for close to two centuries. The earliest microscopes had revealed a previously unknown world of organisms too tiny for the unaided eye to see. The problem was that for a long time, scientists did not realize that some of these microbes cause various diseases. In fact, the general view in those days was that germs were more or less harmless and served no important purpose in nature.

Thus, even though Snow showed that cholera spread as the result of something harmful in certain water sources, most scientists did not yet recognize that germs were the culprit. It was not until the 1860s through the 1880s that a small group of biological pioneers proved the link between certain microbes and a host of deadly diseases. The revelation that germs cause many diseases made it easier for early epidemiologists to track the spread of those maladies because they now knew what to look for. Even so, most medical researchers of the late 1800s and early 1900s continued to search for cures. The first few generations of disease detectives took a different path, however. They worked to determine how various diseases spread. Such knowledge, they believed, would make it easier for medical authorities to predict, control, and maybe even halt some disease outbreaks. And they were correct.

Developing Epidemiological Methods

The early disease detectives found that much of their work could not be done in the confines of a laboratory. Instead, to track down the source of a disease, they often needed to go out into the field—traveling to distant towns, villages, farms, forests, lakes, and other physical settings. There, they could collect water and soil samples and interview the residents of the areas affected by a disease in order to gather clues to solve the mystery of how that sickness spread.

Collecting soil samples and interviewing people are two of the techniques used by early epidemiologists. Each was a tool they could employ to accomplish their work. Over time, they learned to combine these individual tools into complex investigations that they came to call field studies. By the early twentieth century, they had developed three major kinds of studies, and these remain the mainstay of epidemiology today.

The first and perhaps most basic of the three is the case series study, sometimes called a clinical study. Since it was first used in the late 1800s, a prominent physician points out, it has "profoundly influenced the medical literature and continues to advance our knowledge in the present time."[5] A case series study is often inspired by a report of one or more people who recently have become ill and sought help from doctors. If the doctors conclude that their patients have a contagious disease, or if they cannot identify the disease, they will likely ask an epidemiologist to do a case series study. It consists of looking closely at the overall circumstances of the patients.

The principal pieces of information that the disease detectives look for in the study are key factors that most or all the patients have in common. To determine that, the investigators ask a series

field study

A scientific investigation conducted outside of a laboratory setting of questions to find out "what," "when," "where," and "who." The "what" is largely the symptoms, or the diagnosis given by the doctors. The "when" is the approximate day each person became ill. The "where" includes the neighborhood where the patients live, as well as daily routines such as where they recently shopped or ate or visited. The "who" consists of personal details such as gender, age, and type of work of the individual patient and other members of the household.

A Famous Case Series Study

A well-known example of a case series study occurred in Sydney, Australia, in 1941. There an eye surgeon named Norman McAlister Gregg noticed an abnormally large number of cases of babies with eye cataracts. He had seen thirteen in a single year in his own practice alone—a number that seemed unusually high.

Attempting to gather information that might shed light on the issue, Gregg used a tool employed regularly by epidemiologists— the case series study. He devised a series of questions intended

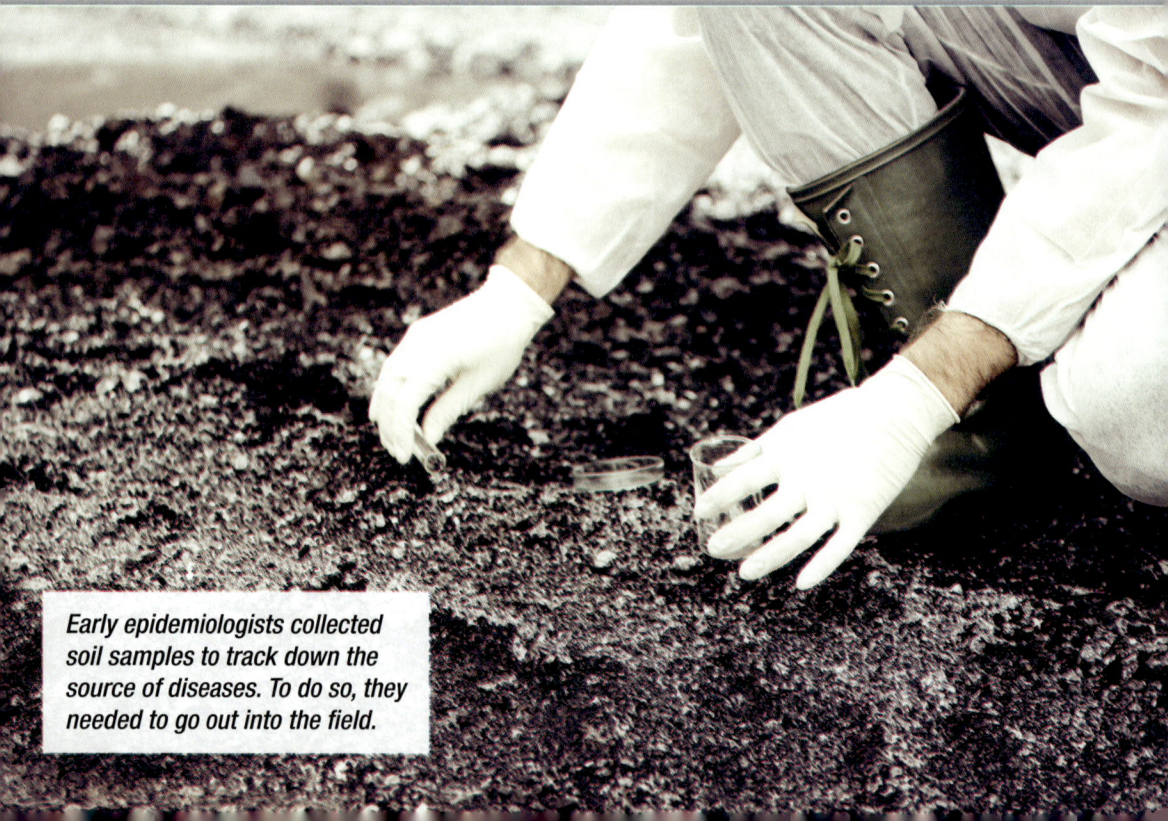

Early epidemiologists collected soil samples to track down the source of diseases. To do so, they needed to go out into the field.

to find out what, if anything, the babies and their mothers had in common. These inquiries asked about various aspects of the mothers' daily routines, the kind of food they ate, their social lives, and so forth. One question related to recent illnesses. That is, had they or someone else in the family been ill in the past few years?

That last question proved vital. Indeed, one factor almost all the women had in common was that they had either been exposed to or contracted rubella, or German measles. From this fact revealed by the study, Gregg suspected something that scientists proceeded to prove—that a fetus in the womb exposed to rubella can suffer certain birth defects, including cataracts.

> **case series study**
>
> A scientific investigation that searches for factors that most or all members of a group of sick people share

How Do Two Groups Differ?

Another major method that epidemiologists employ is the case control study. It consists of a detailed examination of a number of sick people in a given region. The disease detectives try to determine what is different about the members of that group from people in that area who have *not* come down with that sickness. That is, how do the lives and habits of the sick individuals differ from those of the rest? This is another way to reveal how a disease spreads through an area, laying the groundwork for containing the spread.

A case control study conducted by epidemiologist Nathan Shaffer in 1987 offers a striking example. Shaffer sought to help doctors in the small African nation of Guinea-Bissau stop a large cholera outbreak. He first tried to find the main source of the disease. It was well known since John Snow's time that cholera usually spreads through contaminated water. Indeed, Shaffer later recalled, "the epidemic was spreading up and down the coast, [so] right away I suspected shellfish."[6]

Tracking Down a Food-Borne Illness

One of many successful US epidemiological field studies conducted in recent decades occurred in 2004. The Massachusetts Department of Public Health received word of an outbreak of the serious liver disease hepatitis A in Marshfield, a small town located a few miles south of Boston. During the span of only a few weeks, twenty cases of the disease emerged, and local epidemiologists immediately got to work. Knowing that hepatitis A is often caused by eating contaminated food, they interviewed the sick individuals about their daily eating habits. From this data, the investigators suspected that restaurant food was the culprit. But which of the five local Marshfield restaurants served that food? To answer that question, the scientists conducted a case control study to compare the restaurant choices of the sick people to those of locals who did not get sick. Nineteen of the patients answered a special questionnaire, as did thirty-eight healthy people who ate at local restaurants. By comparing the answers given by members of the two groups, the scientists were able to narrow the search down to a single eating establishment. Sure enough, lab tests of the food the restaurant served confirmed that it was the source of the outbreak.

Shaffer was right. But though he had shown how people living on the coast had gotten cholera, he now faced a more difficult mystery. Several people in an inland village who never fished on the coast had also come down with cholera. To find out why, Shaffer used a case control study to compare the recent activities of people on the coast to those of the people in the village. It revealed that one of the villagers had briefly been a dockworker on the coast. That man had died of cholera, and when his body was shipped home, some villagers washed it before burying it. Those same people then prepared the funeral feast. In this way the cholera germs passed from the dead man to several of the villagers.

Long-Term Information Gathering

The third primary type of investigation regularly employed by disease detectives is the cohort study, in which the detectives follow the members of a group of people over time. According to epidemiologists Dag S. Thelle and Petter Laake:

The usual approach is to start with healthy subjects, or subjects without the disease under study. The main purpose is usually to assess the possible effects of different external or internal factors on the risk of disease. Exposure information is collected at baseline for each subject in the cohort. These subjects are followed over time, and the final analysis contains a comparison between those who remained healthy and those who developed the disease under study.[7]

One of the best-known and most successful modern cohort studies is the still ongoing Multicenter AIDS Cohort Study (MACS). Begun in 1984, it originally followed close to six thousand gay and bisexual men, some of whom have since passed away. Over time, disease detectives periodically interviewed the participants, asking dozens of questions about their human immunodeficiency virus (HIV) symptoms (if any), daily habits, and sexual behavior. Much of what science now knows about HIV and acquired immunodeficiency syndrome (AIDS) came from the answers to these questions. According to National Public Radio science reporter Brenda Wilson, "Among the many discoveries that can be attributed to MACS, include basics like how the virus was spreading, how long it took people to get AIDS, and exactly how the immune system failed to protect the body from HIV. It also helped researchers figure how big the epidemic was, particularly in the gay community."[8]

> **virus**
>
> An extremely tiny germ that replicates itself within the cells of the living plant, animal, or person it has invaded

Jumping to Conclusions

The three types of studies are not the only way that epidemiologists identify the origins and spread of various diseases. They sometimes gain such knowledge by correcting and learning from past mistakes or wrong assumptions. A classic case of

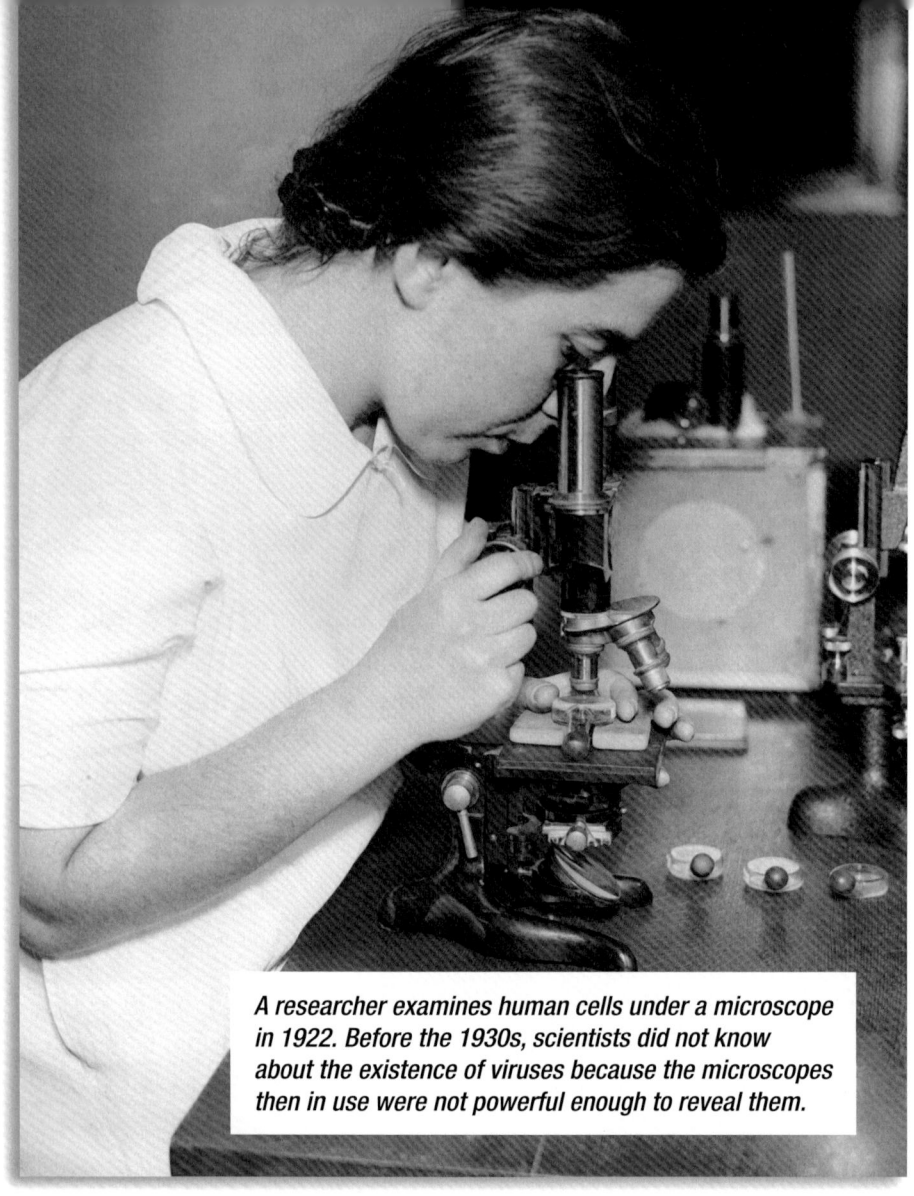

A researcher examines human cells under a microscope in 1922. Before the 1930s, scientists did not know about the existence of viruses because the microscopes then in use were not powerful enough to reveal them.

this process involved early observations of influenza, more commonly known as the flu. Before the 1930s, scientists were unable to conclusively pinpoint what caused the disease and how it spread. The principal problem was that when they used microscopes to examine the bodily fluids of flu victims, no germs were visible. Surely, they reasoned, microbes had to be the culprit. But if so, where were they?

At that point, researchers jumped to two conclusions, one right and one wrong. The right one was that the germs that cause the flu were too tiny to see with the microscopes then in use. The wrong assumption was that those germs were simply smaller versions of the principal disease microbes then known—bacteria. Hence, early epidemiologists tried tracking the flu as if it were a bacterial malady. Not surprisingly, all of those efforts failed.

Finally, in the early 1930s the truth began to come to light. Thanks to the introduction of new microscopes far more powerful than those of the past, scientists found that influenza is caused by a previously unknown kind of germ—a virus. Viruses proved to be many hundreds of times tinier than even the smallest bacteria. Moreover, the researchers found that enormous numbers of viruses exist in bodily fluids such as saliva and mucus. These discoveries led disease detectives to the conclusion that the flu often passes from person to person via droplets of saliva and mucus expelled when someone sneezes, coughs, or even simply exhales.

Proof of the existence of viruses, which infect people differently than bacteria do, opened up whole new vistas for disease detectives. "The story of the discovery of viruses," says Andrew W. Artenstein, a professor at Brown University's school of medicine, "vividly illustrates [periodic major] shifts in scientific thinking, and how these changes lead to new discoveries."[9] Epidemiologists proceeded to combine their increasing knowledge of viruses and other germs with the basic investigatory studies they had developed. This made it possible for them to successfully solve the mysteries of dread contagions like polio, Legionnaires' disease, and Ebola in the decades that followed.

CHAPTER TWO

The Mystery of Sleeping Sickness

In 1903 Scottish-born physician David Bruce—one of the world's first great epidemiologists—inherited a medical mystery. Arriving in Uganda, a nation in east-central Africa then ruled by the British, Bruce led the second of two so-called Sleeping Sickness Commissions sponsored by the prestigious London School of Hygiene and Tropical Medicine. One of the leaders of the first commission, Dr. Cuthbert Christy, greeted Bruce and briefed him on what he had learned in the year he had spent in the region.

First, Christy said, sleeping sickness (known to medical experts as trypanosomiasis) had lived up to its reputation as an extremely deadly and frightening disease. During the first onslaught of its debilitating symptoms, a victim felt tired and developed headaches. Later, he or she was listless and could not function or reason normally. Finally, the victim slept through much of each day but while awake suffered agonizing pain throughout the body. Eventually, the patient lapsed into a coma and perished. Already, Christy told Bruce, many tens of thousands of Ugandans had died from that illness, and there appeared to be no end in sight.

In addition to causing so much misery and death, Christy went on, the disease's assault on human communities had followed a distinct, unusual, and mysterious pattern. "It will be seen at a glance," he explained, that the disease is connected in some way with the great lake [Victoria] or its waters. In no case has the infection spread far inland, 30 or 40 miles being its limit. . . . My observations led me to believe that most cases to be found further than 10 or 15 miles from the lake are cases which have become infected near the shores of the lake. The nearer one approaches the shores of the lake the more prevalent is the disease.[10]

Motivations for Defeating the Disease

That strange pattern of infection repeatedly occupied Bruce's thoughts after he took over for the departed leaders of the first commission. Clearly, he realized, the task of solving this mystery was likely to make an already difficult job even harder. From the start of his tenure in Africa, he was under a great deal of pressure to find a way to end the epidemic and return Uganda to a state of normalcy. The British had taken over that country, along with some other African territories, in 1894, and they were eager to keep the locals healthy and prosperous.

On the one hand, British medical authorities worried about a potentially immense loss of life. Not only might many Ugandans die, but the disease might also spread to Ethiopia, Egypt, and other nearby populous African nations, causing untold death and ruin.

> **trypanosomiasis**
>
> The medical name of sleeping sickness

On the other hand, the British government was strongly committed to reaping the region's large potential economic benefits, including abundant crops, lumber, marble, limestone, salt, copper, nickel, and gold. The British knew that they needed as many able-bodied Ugandans as possible to continually produce those valuable resources. Hence, in the minds of the British, losing enormous numbers of locals was very bad for business.

Bruce saw both sides of the issue. As a physician, he wanted to save as many lives as possible—White and Black. At the same

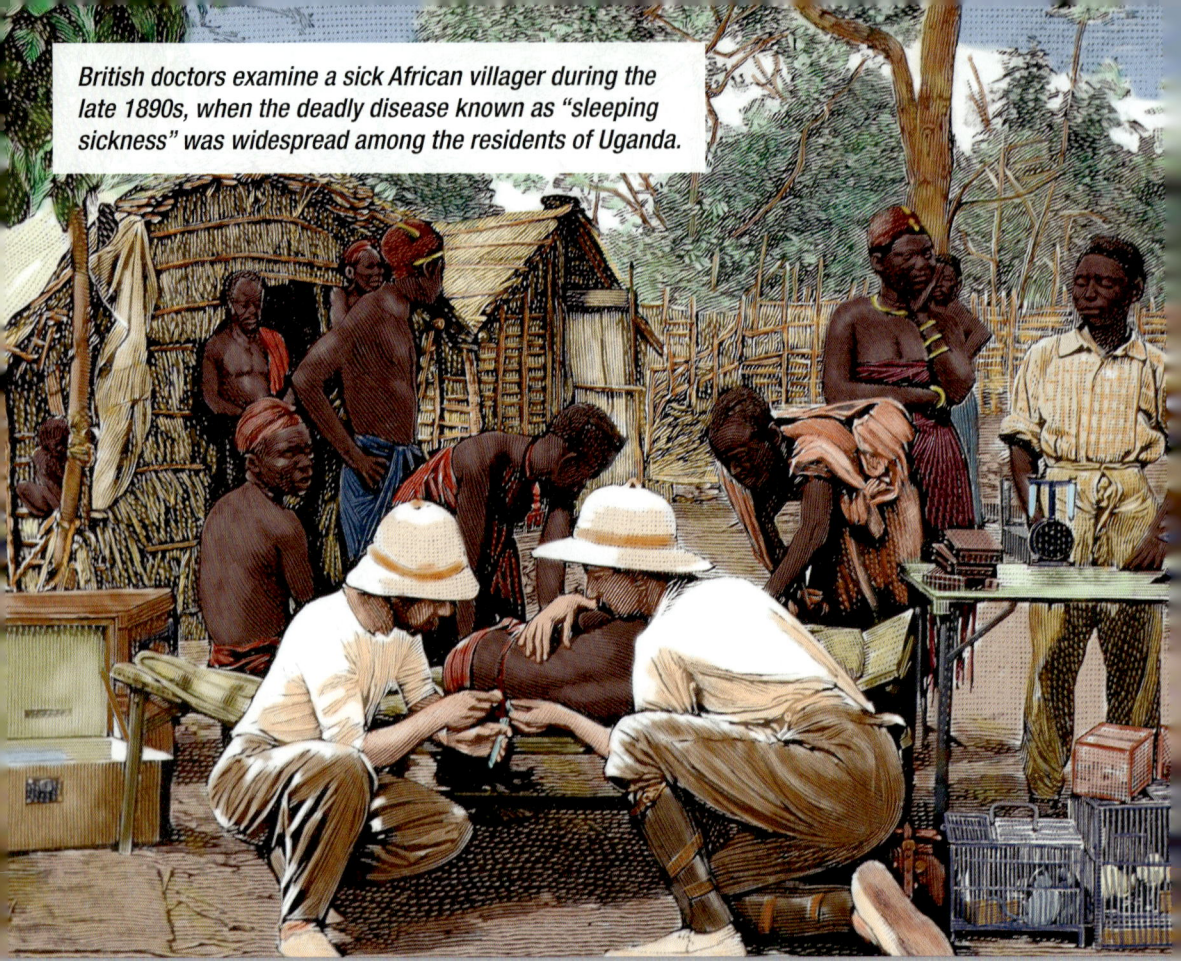

British doctors examine a sick African villager during the late 1890s, when the deadly disease known as "sleeping sickness" was widespread among the residents of Uganda.

time, as a commissioner for the government, he desired to help keep Uganda economically prosperous. However, as a disease detective, he realized—far better than most—that the situation was even more complex and potentially more disastrous than it seemed on the surface.

In particular, Bruce came to see that sleeping sickness, called *lumbe* in parts of Africa, was not a single sickness. Rather, it took a number of forms, some of which did not attack humans. One widespread version of the disease, for instance, affected cattle, horses, and other domesticated animals. In the words of medical researcher Victoria Austin, that version, called *nagama*, had "wide-ranging im-

nagama

A form of sleeping sickness that affects only animals

pacts on socio-economic development in affected regions, including limitation of food supply (meat, milk) and the use of animals in plot cultivation or transport."[11]

The Most Logical Explanation in Doubt

Bruce learned about nagama and other variations of trypanosomiasis partly by touring local villages and, with the help of interpreters, asking many questions. These inquiries collectively form a lengthy, detailed version of a case series study. The more evidence the study gathered, the more apparent it became that all forms of the disease followed the same strange pattern of infection. The victims were almost always residents of villages situated on lake islands, lakeshores, or riverbanks. At the same time, no significant outbreaks of the malady occurred in inland areas.

The most straightforward and logical explanation for this pattern was that dangerous germs must exist in local sources of

From Horse to Scarecrow

Medical researcher David Bruce described the symptoms displayed by a Ugandan horse he encountered suffering from nagama, a form of sleeping sickness that attacks only animals:

> The horse stares. He has a watery discharge from his eyes and nose. Shortly afterwards a slight swelling of the belly and puffiness of the sheath may be noticed, and the animal falls off in condition. The hind extremities also tend to become swollen; and these various swellings fluctuate, one day being less marked, or having disappeared. During this time the animal is becoming more and more emaciated, he looks dull and hangs his head, his coat becoming harsh and thin in places; the mucous membranes of the eyes and gums are pale, and probably slight cloudiness of the cornea is observable. In severe stages, a horse presents a miserable appearance. He is a mere scarecrow, covered by rough hair, which falls off in places. His hind extremities and sheath may be more or less swollen, sometimes to a great extent, and he may become blind. At last he falls to the ground and dies of exhaustion.

Quoted in Tsetse.org, "David Bruce." www.tsetse.org.

water used for drinking, cooking, and washing. This conclusion seemed to fit the scenario established years earlier by John Snow, which is why Christy and his colleagues on the first commission viewed it as the likely answer. And yet there was a problem.

They were unable to find any germs that seemed harmful in the local water samples they tested. Their assumption was that the germs were indeed there but for some reason could not be detected. When Bruce arrived he also tested water samples from Lake Victoria and nearby smaller lakes and rivers. He too could not detect any obviously dangerous microbes. But unlike his predecessors, he doubted that harmful germs were somehow hiding in plain sight.

Instead, Bruce reasoned, the seeming absence of such microscopic culprits suggested that sleeping sickness did not spread through the water itself. It was more likely, he said, that the disease was transmitted by a living thing that dwelled and

Sleeping Sickness Still Lingers in Africa

Although the annual number of cases of sleeping sickness worldwide is today a good deal lower than it was in the late 1800s and early 1900s, the disease remains a threat to poorer Africans in isolated areas of several nations. According to officials of the World Health Organization:

> Sleeping sickness threatens millions of people in 36 countries in sub-Saharan Africa. Many of the affected populations live in remote rural areas with limited access to adequate health services, which complicates the surveillance and therefore the diagnosis and treatment of cases. In addition, displacement of populations, war and poverty are important factors that facilitate transmission. In 1998, almost 40 000 cases were reported, but estimates were that 300 000 cases were undiagnosed and therefore untreated. . . . In 2009, after continued control efforts, the number of cases reported dropped below 10 000 for the first time in 50 years. This decline in number of cases has continued with 997 new cases reported in 2018, the lowest level since the start of systematic global data-collection 80 years ago.

World Health Organization, "Trypanosomiasis, Human African (Sleeping Sickness)," 2020. www.who.int.

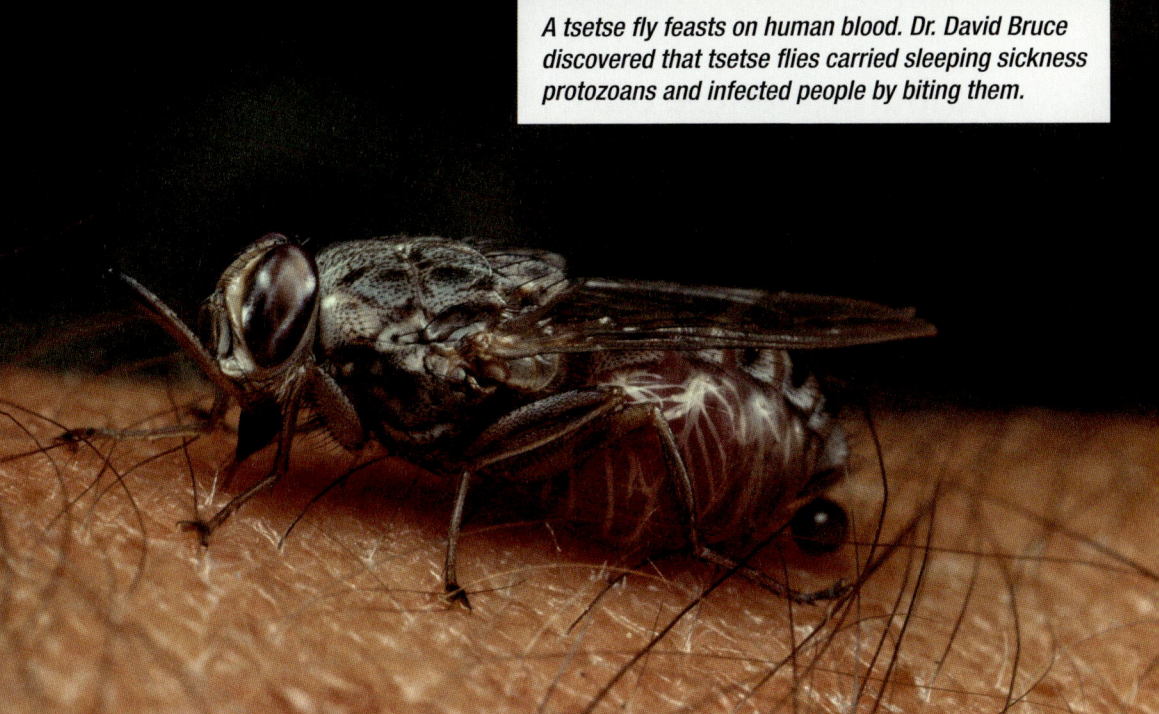

A tsetse fly feasts on human blood. Dr. David Bruce discovered that tsetse flies carried sleeping sickness protozoans and infected people by biting them.

reproduced in and around water. In theory, that creature carried a specific germ that was not harmful to it but was deadly to cattle, horses, and humans.

Bruce's hypothesis turned out to be correct. He showed that the blood of animals suffering from nagama contained tiny protozoan germs that appeared to be causing that ailment. Furthermore, those same microbes existed on the bodies of tsetse flies, bigger versions of ordinary houseflies. When the flies bit an animal or human, Bruce proposed, the protozoans entered the victim's bloodstream, initiating the disease. In his field journal he wrote, "I am of the present opinion that the tsetse fly does play [an important] part in the propagation of the disease. . . . The tsetse acts as a carrier of the living [germ], an infinitely small parasite, from one animal to another, which entering the bloodstream of an animal bitten or pricked, there propagates and so gives rise to the disease."[12]

propagate

To reproduce or spread

To Illuminate the Dark Places

To further confirm his hypothesis, Bruce and his assistants conducted a study of the habits of tsetse flies, as well as the way they were distributed in various parts of Uganda and nearby regions. First, the investigators discovered that those insects reproduced by laying their eggs in water. Second, the flies congregated and bred in the very same areas in which the sleeping sickness epidemics had taken place. It was clearly not a coincidence, the scientists concluded, that these factors overlapped so precisely. Next, Bruce conducted a lab experiment to further demonstrate that flies transmitted the disease's germs to animals and people. Having collected several flies carrying sleeping sickness protozoans, he unleashed them on some lab monkeys. All of the monkeys subsequently contracted the disease.

After proving conclusively that sleeping sickness was a threat to Ugandans who dwelled near water, Bruce pointed out a way to save as many lives as possible. No vaccine or other cure for the disease yet existed. But many people could avoid the flies by moving away from the lakes and rivers. There was initial resistance to that idea among the locals. But in 1907 British officials persuaded most of the villagers in the area to move inland. That bold measure rapidly reduced the incidence of sleeping sickness in Uganda.

Bruce emerged as a hero to many people in both Uganda and Britain. As the late, noted scientist W.J. Tulloch pointed out, it was remarkable that Bruce's "fundamental observations were completed in the short span of only six months. His watchwords were courage, adventure, and service."[13] Like other dedicated disease detectives, Bruce envisioned that such service should be for the good of people everywhere. In a speech Tulloch later gave in England, he stated, "The advance of our knowledge of disease is not for the benefit of one country, but for all—for the lonely African native [who is] dying of Sleeping Sickness . . . as much [as] for the citizens of our own towns. It is the duty of science to go steadily forward, illuminating the dark places in hopes of happier times."[14]

CHAPTER THREE

The Mystery of Polio in the Blood

One day in 1943 Dorothy M. Horstmann, an epidemiologist in Yale University's prestigious medical research lab, noticed something she found unusually puzzling. It was connected to one of that year's three regional US outbreaks of poliomyelitis, or polio (also called infantile paralysis), a disease that causes crippling paralysis, especially in children. The outbreak in question had just occurred in New Haven, Connecticut, where Yale is located. Local authorities urged parents to bring any children who showed physical difficulties to Yale New Haven Hospital to be tested.

Hearing that 111 young people had just been admitted to that facility, Horstmann hurried over to take charge of the blood tests that would be administered. With the help of several nurses, she quickly but carefully collected the samples and took them to her lab for analysis. There she and her colleagues had recently been intensely studying polio, trying to determine how it infected people.

Horstmann found that in the cases of almost all of the children, the tests showed no polio germs in their blood. This did not surprise her. Although it was clear that all had some degree of paralysis and almost certainly did have polio, the microorganisms that cause the disease typically

> **poliomyelitis**
>
> The full medical name for polio

> **paralytic polio**
>
> The most severe form of polio, in which the victim suffers from paralysis

did not show up in victims' blood. They congregated instead in nerve tissues.

What puzzled Horstmann was that one of the 111 children admitted—a nine-year-old girl—*did* have polio microbes in her blood. Moreover, she complained only of a stiff neck and did not appear to have paralytic polio, the form of the illness that leads to paralysis. In fact, Horstmann later pointed out, the girl "would never have been admitted to the hospital if there had not been an epidemic,"[15] which had made her parents overly cautious. Feeling that she may have stumbled onto something significant, Horstmann immediately devoted herself to solving this mystery of polio in the blood. Her instincts in this case were spot on, for she was about to make a discovery that would eventually save the lives of millions of people.

Fighting Bias Before Fighting Disease

The work Horstmann's lab had been doing on polio and the concern that local authorities had shown during the 1943 outbreaks stemmed from widespread fear and worry. In the United States and some other nations, polio had become the most frightening disease of the early to mid-twentieth century. Cases of it had been scattered and relatively few before 1916. In that year it had exploded into epidemic proportions in Brooklyn, New York, and other parts of the northeastern United States. That outbreak killed roughly six thousand people, mostly children, and permanently paralyzed another twenty-seven thousand individuals. Periodic outbreaks had continued to occur in the years that followed.

Scientists in labs across the United States, including the one at Yale, tackled polio with a vengeance, trying to better understand it. The goal was to discover how people contracted it and how it spread through the body to the nerves, where it did most of its damage. It was impossible to find a cure for the disease until the experts understood these things. In the late 1930s and early 1940s, researchers learned a great deal about the disease. It appeared that it entered the body via the mouth, gullet, and stomach and then made its way through the digestive system.

Two major mysteries remained unsolved, however. One was why no polio germs showed up in the bloodstream of the disease's victims. The second burning question was, if the microbes did not travel through the blood, how did they make it from the digestive system to the nervous system?

These were the questions that Horstmann and her colleagues were trying answer in her first year on the Yale team. The work was difficult, but that did not faze her, because she was used to the reality of struggling to achieve positive results. Indeed, becoming a research scientist had been far from easy for her. For many years all of the researchers in Yale's polio unit, as in most other such labs across the country, were men. Horstmann had been forced over the years to deal with male prejudice at almost every turn. In those days most medical schools and labs

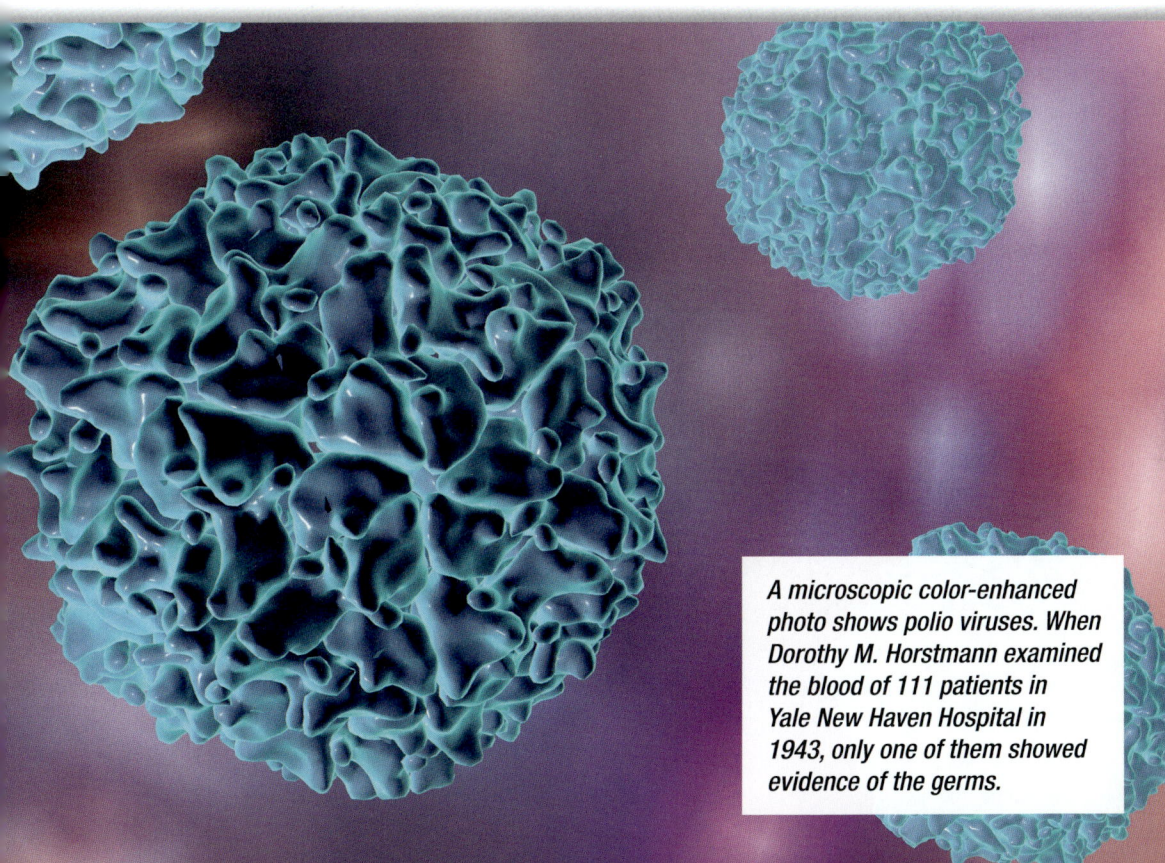

A microscopic color-enhanced photo shows polio viruses. When Dorothy M. Horstmann examined the blood of 111 patients in Yale New Haven Hospital in 1943, only one of them showed evidence of the germs.

excluded women because most assumed that women were not scientifically minded.

Horstmann responded to this bias, in med school and elsewhere, by working twice as hard as her male counterparts. She also made sure that the narrow views held by some people did not dictate her actions. She had a great deal of respect for the work of Dr. John R. Paul, cofounder of Yale's polio research unit. She applied to be part of this group. Paul was immediately impressed with Horstmann and welcomed her to the team. Horstmann plunged ahead into solving the mysteries of polio, work she found to be greatly inspiring. "It had a dramatic immediacy," she later remarked. "When you deal with an epidemic you realize it's an urgent thing. There was so much to be learned."[16]

A History-Making Experiment

Horstmann set to work trying to solve the mystery of the blood samples she had gathered at Yale New Haven Hospital. She needed to know why one girl's blood contained polio germs while

Raising the Money to Fight Polio

The research done on polio in US labs during the 1930s, 1940s, and 1950s was extremely expensive to conduct. Government funding for such research was very rare in those days, so the money had to come from private donations. The biggest of all the private efforts to raise those funds emerged after Franklin D. Roosevelt won his first term as US president in 1932. In the preceding decade he had contracted polio and thereafter required braces, crutches, and a wheelchair to get around. Such setbacks did not deter him from his political ambitions. He served as governor of New York State before winning the presidency.

Inspired by Roosevelt's courage and determination, many Americans began donating money each year to help pay for polio research, and this trend led to the formation of the National Foundation for Infantile Paralysis in 1938. Singer-comedian Eddie Cantor gave that effort the nickname March of Dimes because large numbers of contributors gave a dime to the charity. Over time, the March of Dimes raised tens of millions of dollars and helped make the conquest of the disease possible.

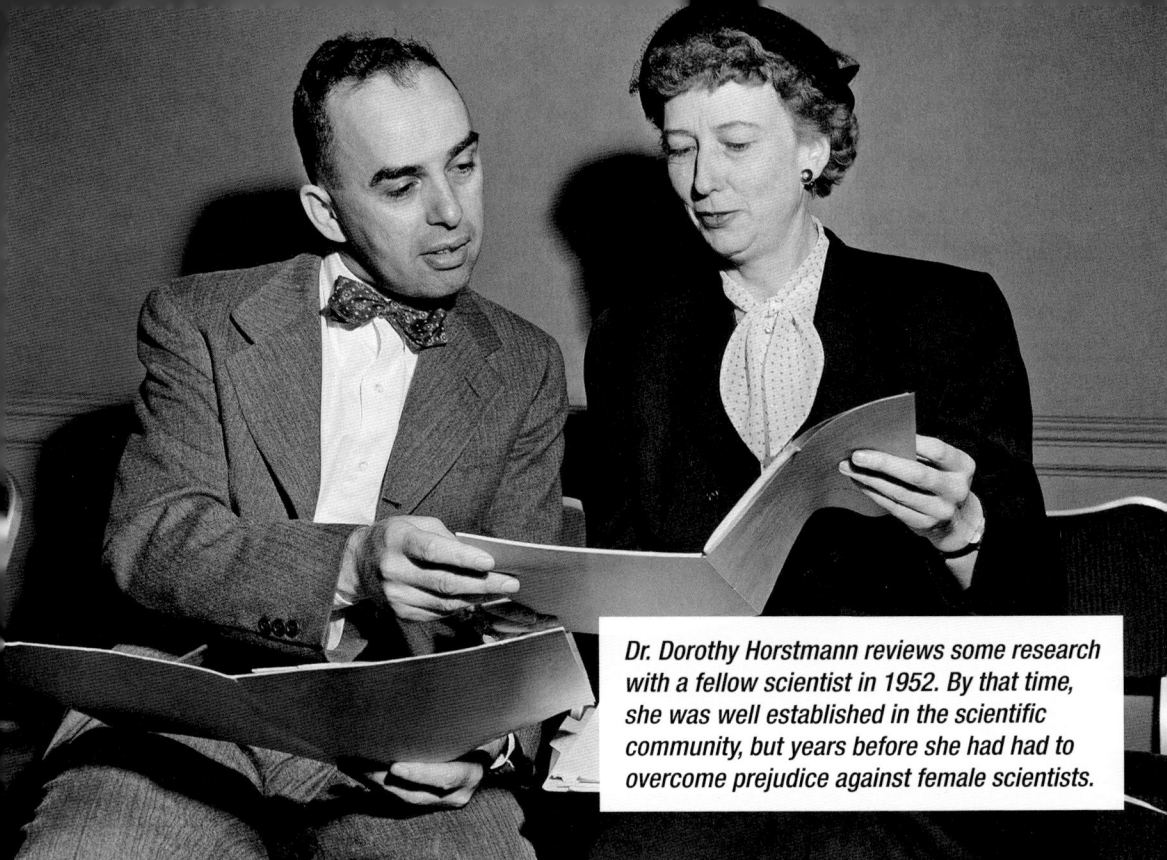

Dr. Dorothy Horstmann reviews some research with a fellow scientist in 1952. By that time, she was well established in the scientific community, but years before she had had to overcome prejudice against female scientists.

the blood of other children who had contracted polio did not. She also wanted to find out why that one girl seemed to have few of the usual symptoms of the disease while the other patients all had varying degrees of paralysis.

Eager to understand this bizarre contradiction, Horstmann began a case series study of the 110 patients whose blood contained no polio germs. The goal was to find out what these young people had in common. She also gathered information relating to the "what?" "where?" and "when?" of the little girl.

It did not take Horstmann long to see that the answer to the riddle was deceptively simple. Moreover, it had been staring her and other researchers in the face for years. The breakthrough came when she determined the "when?" factor for all 111 patients. It showed that the 110 patients with no germs in their blood had had their blood tests after they had developed severe polio symptoms. In contrast, the nine-year-old girl had been tested well before coming down with full-blown symptoms. In fact, other evidence suggested that she had contracted the disease only days before entering the hospital.

Perhaps, Horstmann reasoned, polio microbes were present in the bloodstream only during the brief period between contracting the disease and developing major physical symptoms. Testing that hypothesis would be fairly easy. Wasting no time, she conducted an experiment on monkeys, in which she fed them food containing polio germs and then carefully tested their blood every few hours.

The results of that experiment were history-making. Every single monkey displayed polio microbes in its blood only a couple of days after it ingested the tainted food. Moreover, after a few more days had elapsed, those germs vanished from the bloodstream of each monkey.

Horstmann now saw why she and other researchers had never before seen those germs in tests done on polio victims' blood. They had simply waited too long. That is, blood tests for

The Vaccines Made Possible by Horstmann's Discovery

After disease detective Dorothy M. Horstmann demonstrated how polio spread through the human body, polio research in the United States steadily began to make important strides. It was now possible, for example, to realistically search for a vaccine. The leader of that effort was a young researcher named Jonas Salk. Beginning in 1948, he studied and classified several known strains of polio and, along with other researchers, managed to culture polio germs in the lab. As funding for the research poured in from the March of Dimes and other charities, in 1951 Salk hired over fifty leading scientists. The team worked tirelessly, often logging more than twelve hours a day, six or even seven days a week. By 1953 Salk and his assistants had a preliminary vaccine, which he courageously tested on himself. Mere months later, in April 1954, he directed the vaccination of millions of children aged six to nine. The vaccine proved to be safe and effective, and in April 1955 the US government approved it for distribution on a national scale. Another polio vaccine, developed by researcher Albert B. Sabin, was also approved. Neither vaccine would have been possible without Horstmann's seminal contribution years before.

that malady had traditionally been given only after someone had developed paralysis and sought help from physicians. Well before that stage, Horstmann concluded, the germs had been attacked and killed by soldier cells sent by the immune system. But during that battle a few of the tiny invaders had managed to move on to the nervous system. This neatly explained how polio made the leap from the digestive tract to the nerves; it did so through the bloodstream as one would expect it to.

Praise from Near and Far

Horstmann's epic discovery not only solved the mystery of why so many polio blood tests given over the years had been negative. It also made subsequent preventive measures possible. Researchers attempting to create vaccines to fight polio needed to know exactly how the disease moves through the body. Only then could they pinpoint the optimal time to administer a vaccine.

For her work as a disease detective, Horstmann received well-deserved praise from scientists around the globe. One tribute that she found particularly satisfying came in a private letter from Yale's illustrious historian of medicine, John F. Fulton. Her discovery, he wrote, "is as exciting as anything that has happened in the Yale Medical School since I first came here in 1930 and is a tremendous credit to your industry and scientific imagination." He added, "It is also medical history."[17]

CHAPTER FOUR

The Mystery of the Dead Legionnaires

During the 1976 Christmas holidays, Joseph McDade, an epidemiologist with the Centers for Disease Control and Prevention (CDC), felt particularly frustrated. He had canceled his vacation plans because he was badly needed following the outbreak of a previously unknown disease a few months before. In late July of that year, in Philadelphia, some four thousand members of the Pennsylvania State American Legion, a group of World War II military veterans, had come together to take part in the legion's fifty-eighth yearly convention. In the midst of the festivities, however, a strange illness struck many of them. By the end of August, only a month after the epidemic had begun, 221 attendees had contracted the disease, and 34 of them had died.

The problem was that even as late as the Christmas season, no one had been able to figure out what had caused the outbreak. Twenty disease detectives from the CDC, among them McDade, along with almost one hundred Pennsylvania health care workers, had tackled the mystery. But so far everyone involved in the effort remained baffled.

As the mystery deepened, it was perhaps only natural for the public to speculate about the cause, and some of the theories that circulated tended to be wild, if not ludicrous. Some people proposed that the malady was a bioweapon unleashed by domestic terrorists. Others suggested that it was a Central Intelligence Agency experiment that had gotten horribly out of hand. Still others suspected the epidemic was a cruel hoax intended to make Americans fearful. A few cranks went so far as to blame the outbreak on extraterrestrial invaders testing their advanced weapons on humans.

McDade paid little attention to such unfounded notions. As a scientist, he was confident that the culprit was a disease, and he felt sure that sooner or later, application of old-fashioned medical detective work would reveal its identity. In that effort, he spent nearly every hour of the holiday alone in his lab examining and reexamining slides under his microscope, work that grew tedious and sometimes hurt his eyes. "It's like looking for a contact lens on a basketball court with your eyes four inches above the ground,"[18] he later told reporters.

This hard work eventually paid off, because McDade unraveled the mystery of Legionnaires' disease—an illness whose name did not appear in any medical literature until after it surfaced in July 1976. No less importantly, his discovery quickly led to explanations for several other disease outbreaks. "Sometimes," he later remarked, "what it takes is a large outbreak of a disease to help you discover something that's been percolating for a long time, undetected."[19] His use of the word *percolating* referred to various disease outbreaks that had never been solved. Finally, it became clear that they had been caused by the same illness that had sickened and killed the Philadelphia legionnaires.

One of the CDC's Biggest Cases

At the start of the convention, the members of the Pennsylvania State American Legion were in high spirits as they prepared to celebrate the bicentennial of the birth of the United States. The convention site, the Bellevue-Stratford Hotel, was one of the city's finest lodgings, and more than six hundred of the celebrants had booked rooms there.

The overall positive mood of the participants did not last long, however. On the gathering's second day, some of the legionnaires began to display flu- or pneumonia-like symptoms, including high

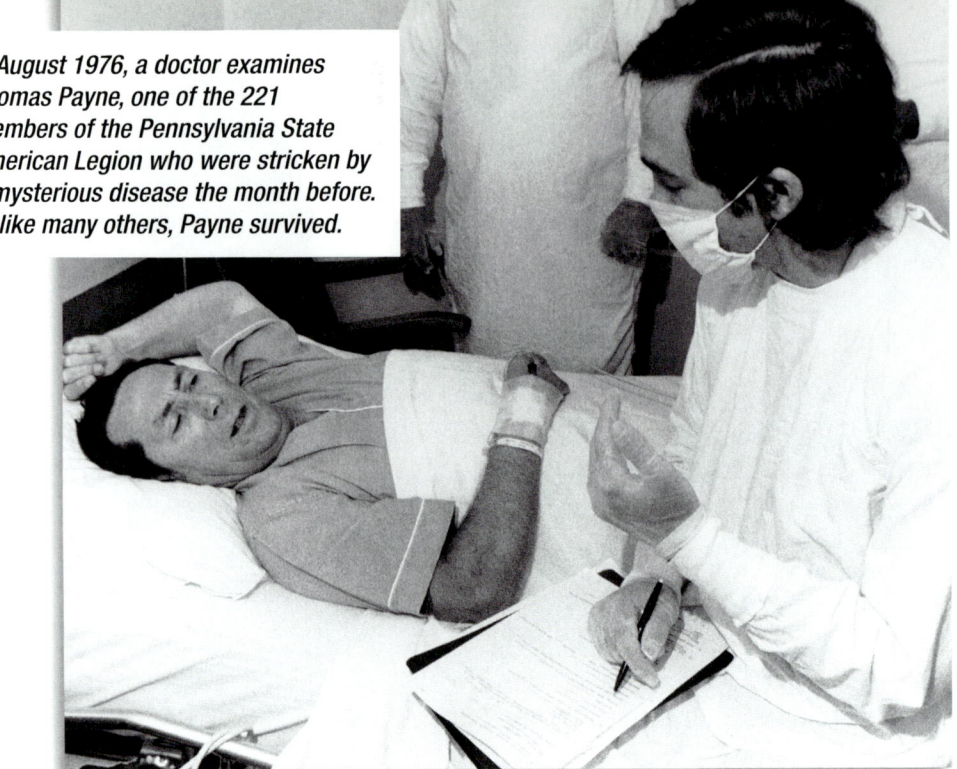

In August 1976, a doctor examines Thomas Payne, one of the 221 members of the Pennsylvania State American Legion who were stricken by a mysterious disease the month before. Unlike many others, Payne survived.

fever, chest congestion, coughing, and trouble breathing. Several others began to display the same symptoms in the two days that followed. Within days one legionnaire had to be rushed to a nearby hospital, where he died.

As both the number of cases and the death toll steadily rose and ordinary flu was ruled out by local physicians, the CDC sent McDade and his colleagues to supplement the work of Philadelphia's own doctors and epidemiologists. Owing to the mysterious nature of the ailment, in short order it had grown into one of the biggest single investigations the CDC had ever launched. One prominent northeastern newspaper reported, "No previous scientific detective effort in history has approached the scale and intensity of the campaign now under way to track down the [Philadelphia disease's] course, source, and pattern."[20]

Correcting a Past Error

In the first few weeks of the investigation, disease detectives conducted case series studies and case control studies. In the process, they conducted thousands of detailed interviews. Initially, one theory was food poisoning. In trying to track down a single food source that might have sickened the legion members, they asked questions about where the members had eaten their meals and what they had eaten. Another theory was that a member had brought a strange new disease with him or her from a distant city. So other questions revolved around prior contacts with people who were showing symptoms of illness.

No solid evidence of these hypotheses emerged, however. From those basic studies, it seemed more likely that some other factor—one located in Philadelphia, or perhaps even in the hotel itself—was involved. That was the supposition that McDade used in his ongoing examination of tissue samples taken from the sick legionnaires.

At first, because of various technical factors, McDade and the other investigators assumed that the microbe that caused the disease was not a bacterium. Instead, most assumed it was a virus. In trying to rule out various illnesses, McDade later recalled, "I noticed every now and again an occasional rod shaped bacterium in some of the tissues, which was considered to be inconsequential. . . . At that point in time I just considered it was an extraneous kind of contaminant."[21]

This assumption was dead wrong. But through perseverance and hard work, McDade ultimately came up with the right answer. During the last few days of 1976, he repeated some steps he had taken before just to be sure. For the second or third time, he examined tissue from a lung of one of the victims and, as before, noticed some rod-shaped bacteria in the mix. This time, however, he did not dismiss them as mere contaminants. Singling them out and scrutinizing them in detail, he concluded that they were a previously unknown variety of bacteria. Moreover, further tests indicated that they were present in the tissues of most of the victims.

bacterium

A common type of microbe, or germ, that is usually rod-shaped, round, or spiral in shape

Legionella pneumophila

The bacterium that causes Legionnaire's disease

McDade and his colleagues soon confirmed that the seemingly stray bacteria actually caused the disease. They also determined the likeliest source of those germs, which the CDC dubbed *Legionella pneumophila*. It appeared that the microbes had grown within and spread outward from the Bellevue-Stratford Hotel's air-conditioning system. There was no way to be sure that this system, which ran throughout the multistory building, could be totally cleansed of the microbes. So health authorities closed down the hotel permanently.

Heroes on the Front Line

The CDC's disease detectives not only managed to solve the mystery of so-called Legionnaires' disease. They also reasoned that the formerly unknown germs involved might have caused one or more past disease outbreaks that remained unexplained. This assumption proved correct. Epidemiologists reopened those older cases and found that *Legionella pneumophila* was indeed the cause in some of them.

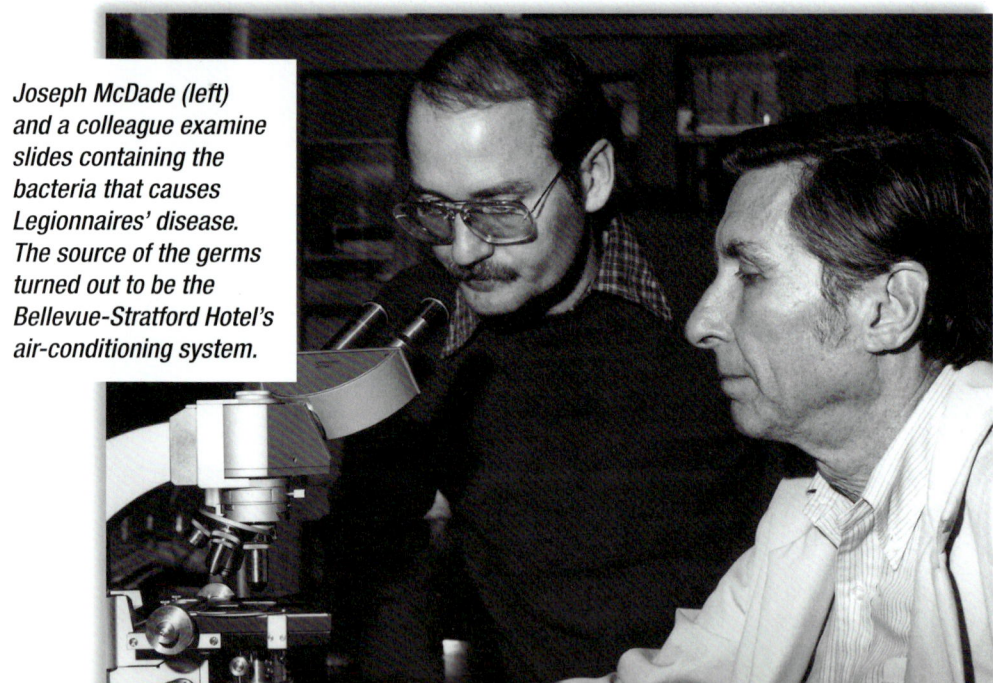

Joseph McDade (left) and a colleague examine slides containing the bacteria that causes Legionnaires' disease. The source of the germs turned out to be the Bellevue-Stratford Hotel's air-conditioning system.

Later Outbreaks of Legionnaires' Disease

Although disease detectives did identify Legionnaires' disease in 1976, there was no way for them to know where that contagion would strike next or when. In fact, the disease has emerged hundreds of times since then, not only in the United States but in other parts of the world too. As summarized by Johnny Denenea, an attorney who specializes in representing victims of Legionnaires' disease:

> At least 250 patients, visitors and employees of the Los Angeles Wadsworth Veterans Administration Hospital succumbed to [it] . . . between 1977 and 1981, before the facility's potable water system was treated with [disinfectant]. From October 10, through November 13, 1989, 33 patients were hospitalized with Legionnaires' disease in Bogalusa, Louisiana. In 1996, in several towns in southwest Virginia, 23 laboratory-confirmed cases of the disease were identified and almost all the victims, when questioned, recalled walking by a display whirlpool spa in a home-improvement store. Other outbreaks were confirmed in foreign countries. In April 1985, 175 patients [contracted the disease and] were admitted to hospitals in Stafford England. . . . [In 1990 an outbreak] at a flower exhibition in the Netherlands caused 318 people to become ill and at least 32 died.

Johnny Denenea, "The History of Legionnaires' Disease," Legionnaires' Lawyer, 2021. https://thelegionnaireslawyer.com.

The investigators showed, for instance, that back in 1957 Legionnaires' disease had badly sickened seventy-eight workers in a meatpacking plant in Austin, Minnesota. The source of the bacteria in that case was the factory's cooling tower. Among the other earlier outbreaks of the disease was one that killed fourteen patients in a psychiatric hospital in Washington, DC, in 1965.

Since the 1970s, disease detectives have also determined that Legionnaires' disease remains a threat. Roughly twenty small-scale outbreaks of it occur each year in the United States alone. But fortunately for the public, the CDC's highly trained investigators can now quickly recognize and treat the disease when it appears. They regularly "risk their lives in defense of public health," medical researcher David Burke points out. "They are the 'front line' against infectious disease, similar to soldiers heading into battle." For that, he adds, they are among society's "unsung heroes."[22]

CHAPTER FIVE

The Mystery of HIV/AIDS

In late 1980 and early 1981, physicians at a hospital in Los Angeles took note of five cases of *Pneumocystis carinii* pneumonia. Often called PCP for short, it is a somewhat rare type of pneumonia caused by a yeast-like microbe. Aware that five cases of it in one place at about the same point in time was highly unusual, the doctors turned to some local medical experts for their opinions. Among them was Michael Gottlieb, a thirty-three-year-old assistant professor at the University of California, Los Angeles, medical school. Like the doctors who had contacted him, he was very concerned. Up until then PCP had been seen almost exclusively in people with weakened immune systems. Typically, this included elderly folk and severely malnourished people.

The five ill patients, however, did not fit this profile. Before developing PCP, all five men were young and healthy. Thus, Gottlieb suspected that their immune systems had been compromised by some previously unknown disease. An added detail that seemed both noteworthy and odd was that all five victims were gay. Whether that had anything to do with their illness was still uncertain. Gottlieb later recalled, "We knew we were on to something."[23] He and the others were just not sure what that something was. It soon became apparent that they would need the help of epidemiologists. So Gottlieb notified the CDC.

The disease detectives sent by the CDC agreed that the mini outbreak of PCP in Los Angeles was extremely unusual. Moreover, they told Gottlieb, the culprit needed to be identified quickly. This was because during the same weeks that the five cases came to light in California, a handful of identical cases—including the fact that all the victims were gay men—had been reported in New York City. The worry was that other cities might harbor similar victims of a new contagion on the verge of sweeping across the country. This suspicion turned out to be correct. The cases in Los Angeles and New York soon proved to be among the first known US cases of AIDS, the disease caused by the human immunodeficiency virus (HIV). It was a deadly illness destined to kill hundreds of thousands of people worldwide.

> ***Pneumocystis carinii* pneumonia (PCP)**
>
> A rare kind of pneumonia caused by a yeast-like microbe

Searching for Key Risk Factors

To prevent or at least contain such a potentially damaging epidemic, the CDC epidemiologists needed to understand how the new disease spread and who in society was most at risk of contracting it. At first, they had little to go on beyond the fact that all the victims they had so far encountered were gay men. The question was whether that was a coincidence or whether sexual orientation factored somehow into the disease and its transmission. Were the risk factors the same for all gay men? Or did the men affected by the disease exhibit specific characteristics or behaviors that other gay men did not?

Trying to explore these questions, in October 1981 the epidemiologists put together a complex case control study. It was designed to examine the risk factors for young, healthy gay men contracting PCP. The investigators reasoned that those in that group who had a high risk of catching PCP also likely had a high risk of

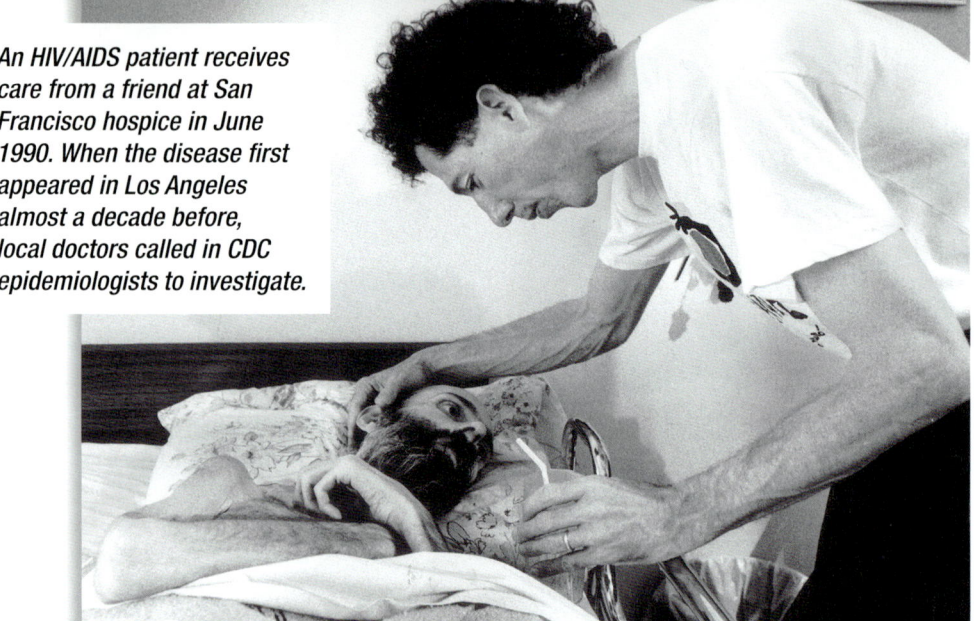

An HIV/AIDS patient receives care from a friend at San Francisco hospice in June 1990. When the disease first appeared in Los Angeles almost a decade before, local doctors called in CDC epidemiologists to investigate.

getting the mystery disease. Clearly, the latter had compromised immune systems and left them open to acquiring PCP in the first place. Thus, the study compared the gay men who had contracted PCP to gay men who had not contracted it. The investigators made sure that the men in the control group—those who had not become ill—were the same age and lived in the same cities as the victims.

The study showed that the young men who had gotten PCP did have higher risk factors than their counterparts who had avoided the disease. One of the biggest of those factors was that the disease's victims had tended to have numerous sexual partners each year, whereas those who had had only one or two sexual partners had not gotten sick. That indicated that having multiple sexual partners seriously increased the chances of contracting the disease. Another significant risk factor the study revealed was exposure to fecal matter during anal sex. Thus, the gay men who regularly engaged in anal intercourse were more at risk of becoming ill than those who rarely or never engaged in it.

Other Ways of Contracting the Disease

The disease detectives had solved part of the mystery of how the new ailment spread; namely, through certain risky behaviors. One of the authors of the initial CDC study stated, "Although the cause of the [impairment of the immune systems of] homosexual men remains unknown, the study presented here . . . has identified a distinctive lifestyle as an important risk factor."[24]

This turned out to be only part of the story, however. Not long after conducting this initial study, other victims of the new disease emerged—and many were not gay or male. Further studies showed that the illness could be contracted through blood transfusions or when drug addicts shared needles. Also, it was found that pregnant women could pass the illness to their unborn child. These discoveries indicated that the new disease had nothing to do with simply being gay. Rather, it appeared that a microbe of some kind passed from person to person—any person—through blood and semen and that gay men had merely been the first victims to come to light. The CDC confirmed these facts by conducting cohort studies of the different groups of victims in the years that followed. Those groups included needle-using drug addicts, pregnant women, and people who had received blood transfusions.

As these studies continued, teams of microbiologists and other biomedical researchers hunted for the offending microbe

The Continuing Mystery of Robert Rayford

Although the US HIV/AIDS epidemic emerged in Los Angeles and New York City in 1980–1981, at least one case of HIV appeared much earlier in a spot far from those cities. In 1968 a fifteen-year-old boy named Robert Rayford was admitted to a St. Louis, Missouri, hospital with what appeared to be a mystery illness. Very weak, emaciated, and riddled with cancerous skin sores, he was close to death and in fact did die a few months later, in May 1969. No one at the time had any inkling that Rayford was suffering from AIDS, the disease caused by the HIV virus, because both the virus and the disease were then unknown. Fortunately for medical science, two of the doctors working at the hospital collected some of his tissue samples and froze them. Years later, in 1985, one of those physicians sent the samples to a lab that was testing human tissue samples for HIV. The samples appeared to match all the criteria for HIV, prompting various experts to call it the earliest known case in the United States. To this day, however, epidemiologists lack enough evidence to show exactly how the boy contracted the disease.

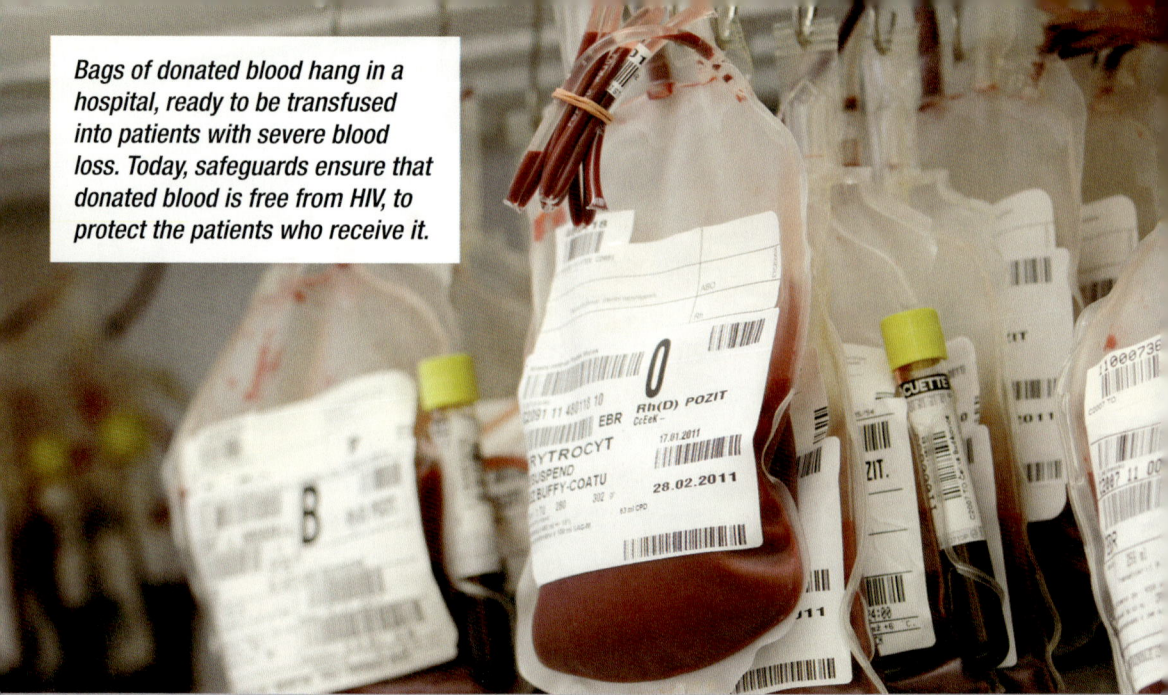

Bags of donated blood hang in a hospital, ready to be transfused into patients with severe blood loss. Today, safeguards ensure that donated blood is free from HIV, to protect the patients who receive it.

itself. The hope was to find it as quickly as possible because the disease was spreading rapidly, infecting tens of thousands of people. (It was destined to become the leading cause of death for Americans aged twenty-five to forty-four by 1995.) One of the teams searching for the contagion, led by Robert C. Gallo of the University of Maryland, did manage to identify it with relative speed. Announcing the discovery in 1984, at first Gallo and the others called it HTLV-III (for human T-cell lymphotrophic virus, type 3), but in 1986 they renamed it HIV.

Another HIV Mystery to Solve

Gallo and his colleagues received widespread praise for their work in identifying the virus. But they had no way of knowing the answer to a question that reporters and others repeatedly asked them: where had the virus come from? Tracking down the origins of HIV/AIDS was the job of epidemiologists, some of whom tackled that mystery in the late 1980s and early 1990s.

For this sort of specialized work, which seeks answers from the world of the past, disease detectives cannot employ their usual case and cohort studies. Instead, they delve into the microscopic world of genes, the tiny particles that determine the structure of all living things. As a virus like HIV evolves, it changes slightly over time, just as humans, animals, and plants do. The disease detectives therefore aimed to compare the genetic structure of modern HIV to that of much older samples of the virus. Those samples came from scattered preserved human remains from the 1800s and early 1900s. According to University of Arizona scientist Michael Worobey, "By studying differences in the viral [genes], scientists estimate how long it has been since the [most recent versions] could have diverged from a common source."[25]

> **genes**
>
> The tiny particles within living cells that determine the structure of plants, animals, and people

These studies were revealing. By 1994 it had become clear that a version of HIV existed in the 1800s in wild populations of chimpanzees and gorillas in West Africa. When people of that period captured those primates and slaughtered them for meat, the hunters were contaminated by the nonhuman blood, which contained the viruses. From there, over the course of decades, the HIV microbes spread slowly but steadily around the globe. As they did so, they continued to evolve and change until taking a particularly lethal form in the late twentieth century.

> **genomic epidemiology**
>
> The relatively new branch of epidemiology that studies the origins and evolution of disease-causing microbes

The ability to track changes in the genetic structure of disease germs has added a crucial new addition to disease detectives' tool kit. A few of these investigators now specialize in this sort of work, which is known as genomic epidemiology. As one scientist puts it, they and their studies are significantly increasing human knowledge about "how and why infectious diseases spread. As these genomics-based methods continue to improve in speed, cost, and accuracy, they will be increasingly used to inform and guide infection control and public health practices."[26]

CHAPTER SIX

The Mystery of Deadly Ebola in Africa

When Australian epidemiologist Katrina Roper first visited the small West African nation of Sierra Leone in 2014, she found that the work she had come to do was more difficult than she had imagined. The Australian National University had sent her there to work with an international team of disease detectives who were desperately trying to contain an outbreak of Ebola. That highly infectious viral illness, which nearly always kills its victims, is characterized by symptoms such as fever, fatigue, vomiting, diarrhea, and liver failure. This frightening disease had first appeared on a small scale in Africa in 1976. Later, in the 1990s, a bigger outbreak had occurred on that continent. An even larger outbreak emerged in 2014. That outbreak lasted almost two years and infected almost thirty thousand people in three countries—Sierra Leone, Guinea, and Liberia.

What initially frustrated Roper was that many of the local people seemed unaware of how Ebola spread. Many continued to engage in their normal activities without taking precautions, even as the number of people afflicted with the disease rose. Typical was an incident in which Roper tried to find a villager who had recently come into contact with an Ebola victim. She wanted to warn the villager that he had been exposed to the disease, as well as to keep him from infecting others. When she reached his village, she was disturbed to hear that he was about to throw a large engagement party at his home. Such an event was likely to cause the malady to spread throughout the local area.

Thus, Roper found that her job was not only to track the spread of the disease. She learned that another aspect of an epidemiologist's job is to educate local populations on how to avoid risky behaviors that tend to increase transmission of a given sickness. Yet this was no easy task, she discovered. First, she had to get the locals to trust that she—a stranger—was not there to exploit or judge them. "You know," she later recalled, "I'm a foreigner coming into their country and I'm asking a lot of personal questions and I'm being very persistent and that can really be quite confronting for the person being questioned. So we'd spend a lot of time trying to explain why it was important to find out all the information and point out that no one was in trouble for being sick."[27]

The Price Paid for a Wrong Assumption

In time Roper was able to gain the trust of the local people she dealt with. That made doing her primary task much easier. That task was to help contain the outbreak by determining how it was spreading in that particular region at that specific time. To accomplish that goal, she and other disease detectives working in West Africa employed a combination of methods. The first of those was the tried-and-true epidemiological approach of doing case studies that involved asking lots of questions. Describing the case series studies she did in small towns, Roper later said that in large part it consisted of "literally walking the streets. We were just looking for people who might be sick, talking to people, just gathering information. It really is detective work. And as you gather information you find out who might have moved into an area, who's left an area, who's feeling sick, and you of course would be looking for any dead bodies."[28]

Although this method of investigation was essential and definitely helped guide the epidemiologists and other medical personnel, complications arose. The biggest of these obstacles was

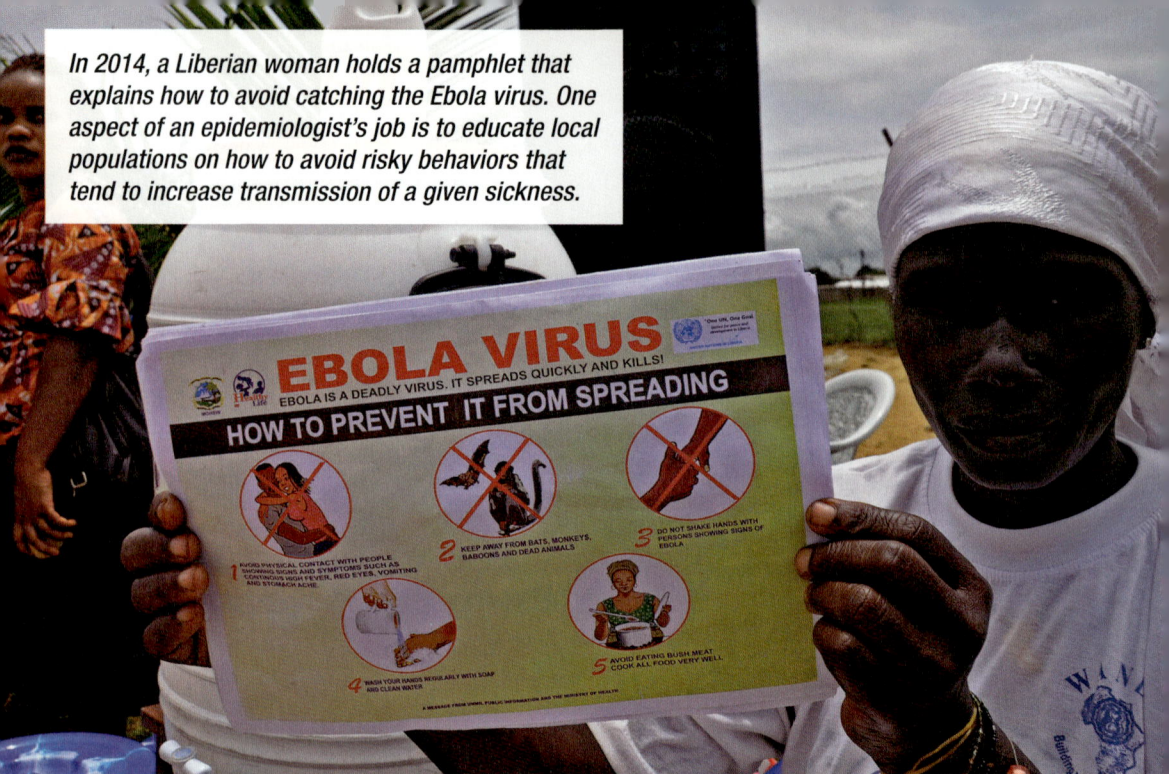

In 2014, a Liberian woman holds a pamphlet that explains how to avoid catching the Ebola virus. One aspect of an epidemiologist's job is to educate local populations on how to avoid risky behaviors that tend to increase transmission of a given sickness.

that the outsiders had arrived in Sierra Leone, Liberia, and Guinea with certain preconceived notions. A major one was the assumption that the local people—mostly rural farmers—would behave like rural farmers in other parts of the world. In particular, the investigators reasoned, the vast majority of rural folk, being tied to the land, would likely remain in and around their villages most of the time. That would, in turn, tend to keep the Ebola virus from readily spreading to other regions.

But as it turned out, this assumption was incorrect. The people of that region of West Africa were far more mobile that rural farmers tended to be in other parts of the world. The price of a wrong assumption like this can be high. And it was. The disease spread much farther and faster than anticipated by the scientists. University of British Columbia scholar Tom Koch explains:

> Nobody realized until too late that the [initial cases of the disease] occurred among . . . [an] indigenous rural population whose members regularly visited similar villages

across porous, unmanned national borders (Guinea, Liberia, Sierra Leone). Assuming a localized outbreak, disease experts did not anticipate the travel patterns that existed between a set of [local] villages on the one hand and, on the other, villagers' regular travel to and from the large, coastal cities of all three countries. For their part, villagers did not perceive until too late that deaths in villages kilometers away might be causally related to those occurring weeks later in their home villages. The potential for early containment [of Ebola] was lost as a result.[29]

Using Every Available Tool

The main problem was that in the initial months of the epidemic, before the epidemiologists realized how mobile many of the local people actually were, those investigators did not ask some of the questions they should have in their case studies. As a result, the studies did not always reflect the population movements that regularly occurred. Moreover, even when the scientists did begin asking the right questions, they faced another difficulty. It was that the weekly travel patterns of thousands of villagers were highly complex and difficult to pin down simply by asking questions.

The investigators managed to solve that problem by using specialized maps to supplement the interviews employed in the case studies. Teams of interviewers went to numerous isolated farms and villages and asked the residents to describe where they had gone, which roads or paths they had taken, and how often they had traveled. With this information and with photos of the area taken by cameras in orbiting satellites, the epidemiologists constructed the maps. These visual guides helped them track the many and complex ways that Ebola spread both within each country and from country to country.

localized

Limited or restricted to a given area or region

mutation

A slight change in the genetic structure of a plant or animal

As this work was going on, other disease detectives attempted to track Ebola's spread by studying the virus's genes. They knew that viruses mutate, or change their genetic make-up over time. This typically happens as the virus moves from one host to another; it adapts to each new host by making very slight changes. The genomic epidemiologists reasoned that looking for mutations could help them trace the disease's spread.

If, for example, they found one form of the virus in place A and the same form of it 50 miles (80 km) away in place B, they would know that it could not have spread slowly through several hosts. They would know this because if it had spread slowly through several hosts, there should have been slight but measurable mutations along the way. If the virus was the same in both places, therefore, it meant that a person carrying the virus had traveled from place A directly to place B and infected someone there.

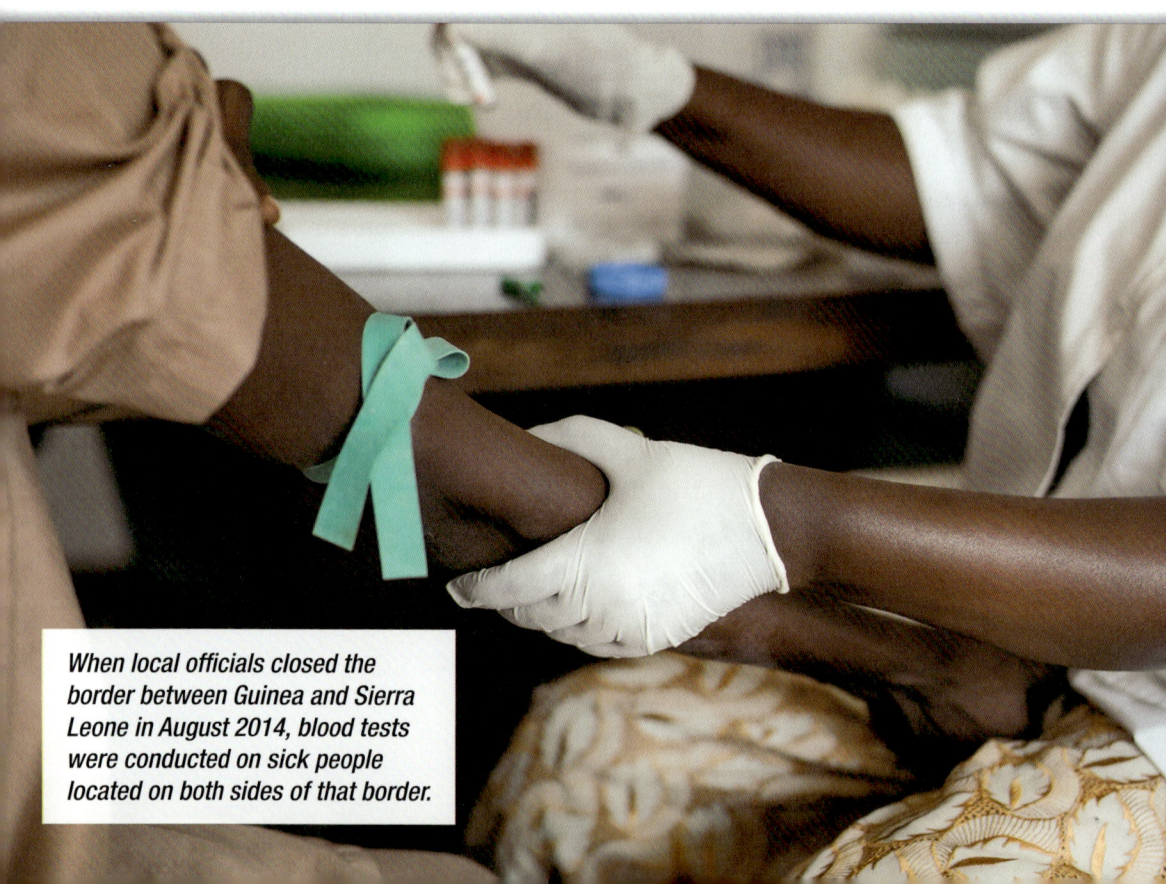

When local officials closed the border between Guinea and Sierra Leone in August 2014, blood tests were conducted on sick people located on both sides of that border.

An Insider's View of Tracking Ebola

The job of tracking a deadly infectious disease such as Ebola can be exhausting, both physically and emotionally. It requires persistence and fortitude. Australian epidemiologist Katrina Roper recalls some of the challenges of conducting fieldwork in the West African nation of Sierra Leone during the 2014–2016 Ebola outbreak.

> I don't think anything really prepares you for the first time you see a lot of bodies lying on the side of the road or the first time you watch a group of people walking down the road and then coming into a clinic because someone's sick and then all of a sudden that person just collapses and they just lose consciousness. You know, seeing such vast numbers of sick people and dead and dying people [from a scary disease like Ebola] is really very [challenging]. I think for me keeping strong meant that I had to look after myself first in terms of making sure I did eat and drink properly, make sure I got some sleep. . . . [Mostly] it was just a lot of work. You just have to keep focussing [on the idea] that it's all for the betterment of the country.

Quoted in Madeline Short, "WorldLink: The 'Disease Detective' on Ebola's Case," Australian Centre for Health Security, 2019. https://indopacifichealthsecurity.dfat.gov.au.

This kind of knowledge came in handy by showing the investigators whether specific attempts to contain the disease were working. When officials closed the border between Guinea and Sierra Leone, for instance, blood tests were conducted on sick people living on both sides of the border. When a largely unaltered form of the virus was found on both sides, it became clear that at least a few people had managed to sneak across the border undetected.

As an epidemiological tool, genetic studies proved a valuable addition to other tools, including traditional case studies and special maps, during the 2014–2016 outbreak. Using the full arsenal of possible methods appears to be the wave of the future for disease detectives examining exotic new contagions, says leading Ebola researcher Peter Piot. To successfully attack and defeat those threats, he states, "we must use every possible approach and tool available."[30]

CHAPTER SEVEN

The Mystery of the Virus from Wuhan

In December 2019 the deadly COVID-19 microbe, a new type of coronavirus, quietly and ominously began to spread outward from its original location—Wuhan, China. At the time, Tyler Shelby was on his way to becoming a professional disease detective. Then in his mid-twenties, he had almost completed his degree in epidemiology at Yale University, in New Haven, Connecticut.

Part of Shelby's reason for choosing that career path was that he was a huge fan of the great fictional detective Sherlock Holmes and his faithful sidekick, Dr. Watson. Shelby envisioned himself applying the same kind of cleverness displayed by those sleuths to the task of tracking the spread of modern diseases. He often told family and friends that he wanted to become an expert in "shoe-leather epidemiology," a term coined in recent years by Vermont health official Daniel Daltry. ("Shoe-leather" is a colorful adjective long applied to old-style detectives who relentlessly walked the streets searching for clues.)

When COVID-19 expanded into a global pandemic in the early months of 2020, Shelby felt called to go out and combat it despite his not yet having his degree. Gathering advice from some of his professors and other professional epidemiologists, he organized a team of a few dozen like-minded amateur investigators. The goal was to help the professionals with contact tracing. Essentially, it is a slight variation of the basic epidemiological case series study, in which the investigators ask many detailed questions about "where," "when," and "who." One of those questions is inevitably, "Who did you recently come into close contact with?" Depending on the answer, the contact tracer adds one more step to the process. He or she contacts the persons the interviewee named and warns them that they may have been exposed to a disease. The hope is that those contacts will isolate themselves, thereby slowing the spread of that illness.

> **contact tracing**
>
> A version of a case series study in which the investigator contacts people exposed to a disease and warns them to quarantine themselves

Shelby and his fellow amateur sleuths tracked down people in this manner almost day and night for months. Over time, however, they conceded that they could only do so much. As the number of COVID-19 cases in the United States continued to skyrocket, they realized that they were steadily being overwhelmed. They were not surprised, because they had recognized early on that this could happen if the pandemic grew big enough. Nevertheless, they decided that in spite of their limitations, they would continue with the work. Shelby later recalled, "From the beginning one of our [repeated slogans] was: 'We'll do as much as we can for as long as we can.' Everything was unclear and nobody knew what was around the corner. We just accepted that uncertainty. We figured that we're not going to be able to resolve everything, but we're going to do what we can."[31]

Disease Detectives Confront the Contagion

Indeed, the sheer scope of the COVID-19 pandemic severely challenged everyone who had any part in trying to understand and control its spread. By early March 2021, globally the virus had infected nearly 116 million people and killed almost 2.6 million; that included roughly 29 million cases and 520,000 deaths in the United States, according to the Johns Hopkins University Coronavirus Resource Center.

Nevertheless, experts everywhere agree that had it not been for epidemiologists from a number of nations, these frightening figures would likely have been far higher. When the virus first emerged in east-central China, the manner in which it spread, its degree of infectiousness, and who in society was most vulnerable to it were largely unknown. The best ways of avoiding and treating it were therefore also uncertain. Determining these things was the chief goal of the many epidemiologists who stepped forward to confront the contagion.

The first disease detectives on COVID-19's case were the approximately eighteen hundred epidemiologists assigned by the Chinese government to help contain the outbreak in Wuhan. They quickly traced the outbreak to one of that city's live food markets, where infected meat was apparently the source of the virus. They also quarantined large numbers of local citizens, a move that ultimately kept the disease from decimating the Chinese heartland. In addition, the Chinese investigators used case series studies, case control studies, and other tools, which determined two im-

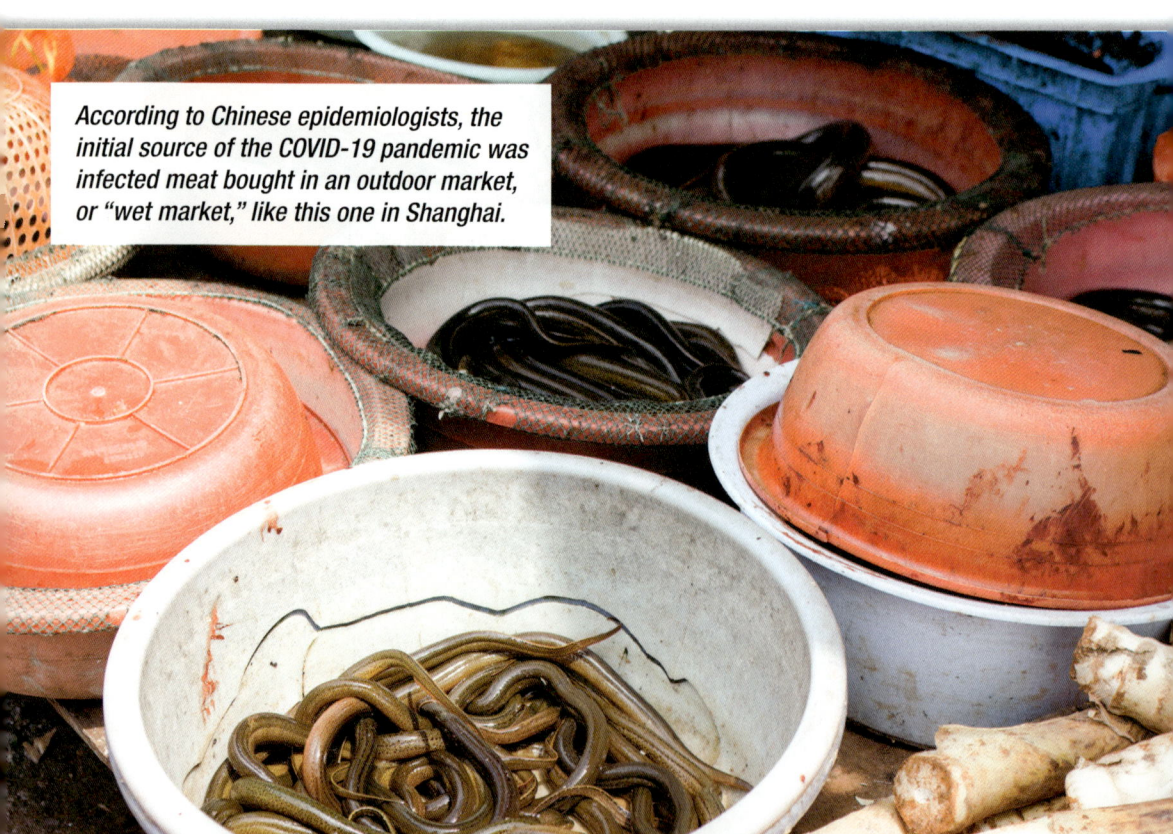

According to Chinese epidemiologists, the initial source of the COVID-19 pandemic was infected meat bought in an outdoor market, or "wet market," like this one in Shanghai.

Studies Show That Masks Reduce Spread

Several CDC-sponsored epidemiologists were among the disease detectives who studied the effectiveness of mask wearing to avoid contracting the virus that causes COVID-19. Among the epidemiological studies that concluded that masks did indeed help reduce transmission were case control studies of various kinds. One conducted by CDC investigators, in conjunction with the Thai Ministry of Public Health, was reported to the public in November 2020. Conducted largely during the preceding April, the study compared people who wore masks to people who did not wear them. What made it a valid comparison is that the study followed up on and interviewed more than one thousand people who attended various crowded public events, including a boxing match. Some did get sick with the disease, while members of a larger group did not. Of the participants who came down with symptoms of the disease, most did not wear masks at any of the events. In contrast, most of those who did wear masks did not get sick. "Our findings provide evidence supporting consistent mask-wearing . . . to reduce transmission in public gatherings."

Quoted in Pawinee Doung-ngern et al., "Case-Control Study of Use of Personal Protective Measures and Risk for SARS-CoV 2 Infection, Thailand," Centers for Disease Control and Prevention, 2020. wwwnc.cdc.gov.

portant factors. The first was that people aged sixty and over had a higher risk of becoming very ill from the virus than younger people did. Second, mask wearing and moderate social distancing appeared to reduce the sickness's spread, although to what extent remained somewhat unclear.

Epidemiologists in Europe, the United States, and elsewhere wanted to confirm these findings. At first they had a limited amount of patient data to work with. But that situation swiftly changed as the weeks progressed and increasing numbers of cases were reported around the globe. With more and more data available, case studies, coupled with physical exams of the those infected, allowed investigators to establish an alarming fact. Namely, the virus could be transmitted by people showing no symptoms; that

social distancing

The act of maintaining 6 feet (1.8 m) or more between oneself and others in order to avoid transmission of disease microbes

Another Benefit of Masks

Studies of mask wearing have revealed a benefit beyond reducing the risk of contracting the coronavirus that causes COVID-19. "Masking may not only protect you from infection but also from severe illness," explains Monica Gandhi, an infectious disease expert at the University of California, San Francisco. The studies indicate that mask wearing decreases the number of individual germs the wearer might absorb from someone who is infectious. Fewer germs, Gandhi explains, may mean less severe illness even if the person ends up contracting the virus. "It's another argument for masks," says University of Edinburgh scientist Paul Digard.

Quoted in Lynne Peeples, "Face Masks: What the Data Say," *Nature*, October 6, 2020. www.nature.com.

is, by people who were merely carriers. That meant that the disease had the potential to spread quickly and quietly through local populations. "Taken together," say the editors of the prestigious scientific journal *Nature*, "these studies helped to alert many governments to the fact that the situation might be much more severe than they had anticipated. The findings suggested that hospitals worldwide needed to prepare for a high number of admissions to intensive care."[32]

Lockdowns and Masks

As COVID-19 continued to spread rapidly, epidemiologists' warnings proved valid. Hospitals in numerous countries found their intensive care units swamped with patients needing respirators, since one of the disease's chief symptoms is difficulty breathing. At the same time, disease detectives everywhere were trying to discern the best ways of stopping, or at least slowing, transmission of the virus.

One approach was to lock down various public venues where large numbers of people gathered. The Chinese had locked down Wuhan in January 2020 and done the same with dozens of other cities the following month. This had proved effective in reducing the spread of COVID-19, and not long afterward European, Canadian, Australian, and US epidemiologists advised their governments to do the same. As a result, many schools were closed. Also, large public gatherings, including major sporting events—the 2020 Summer Olympics in Tokyo among them—were canceled.

Disease detectives also conducted numerous case studies that confirmed Chinese investigators' preliminary findings about the effectiveness of masks and social distancing. Both did in fact slow the virus's spread.

Ongoing Expansion of Epidemiology

These and the many other studies of COVID-19 conducted by epidemiologists did more than change public behavior and thereby save lives. The pandemic was so enormous and its negative effects so far-reaching that it forever changed the nature of the science of epidemiology itself. Most notably, medical experts say, that discipline expanded, becoming more multidisciplinary. According to the editors of Nature, there was a large influx of researchers from other fields, among them mathematics, physics, and computer science. This reliance on ideas and data from other sciences does not "diminish the impact of epidemiology,"

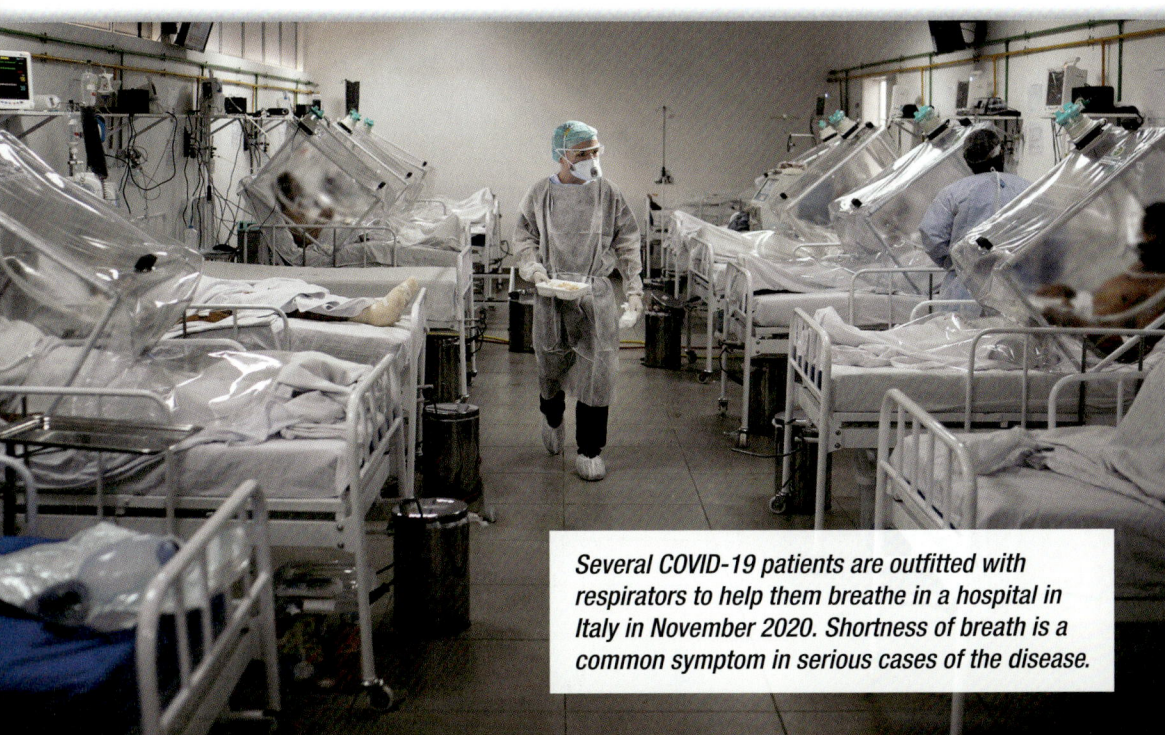

Several COVID-19 patients are outfitted with respirators to help them breathe in a hospital in Italy in November 2020. Shortness of breath is a common symptom in serious cases of the disease.

the editors suggest. Rather, it conjures up the image of a brighter, more disease-free future, in which there is "continuous and transparent conversation between researchers, policymakers and the public."[33]

The disease detectives themselves, Harvard University epidemiologist Marc Lipsitch among them, were happy to receive that extra input from other scientists. "Done well," he says, "epidemiology synthesizes many branches of science using many methods, approaches, and forms of evidence. No one can be expert in all of these specialties . . . [and] a scientist should be open to learning about all of these kinds of evidence and more. . . . We should use every possible source of insight at our disposal to gain knowledge."[34]

As any epidemiologist will admit, however, it is not only the knowledge itself that called him or her to the profession. It was also the adventurous aspect of tracking down clues, some of them extremely difficult to find, in order to uncover that knowledge. As former epidemiologist Seema Yasmin puts it, "There's the thrill of chasing mysterious microbes, identifying patient zero [the first victim] in an outbreak, and the lifelong friendships that are formed along the way."[35]

> **patient zero**
>
> In an epidemic or pandemic, the first person to contract the disease

SOURCE NOTES

Introduction: Birth of a New Medical Science

1. Quoted in Judith Summers, *Soho: A History of London's Most Colorful Neighborhood*. London: Bloomsbury, 1989, p. 113.
2. Quoted in Peter Vinten-Johansen, "In Fairness to Snow," John Snow Archive and Research Companion, October 19, 2013. http://johnsnow.matrix.msu.edu.
3. Addison Brickson, "John Snow and Epidemiology," ArcGIS Online. www.arcgis.com.
4. Quoted in Ralph R. Freriches, "Reverend Henry Whitehead," UCLA Department of Epidemiology. www.ph.ucla.edu.

Chapter One: Disease Detectives' Basic Methods

5. Mohammad H. Murad et al., "Methodological Quality and Synthesis of Case Series and Case Reports," *BMJ Evidence-Based Medicine*, April 2018. https://ebm.bmj.com.
6. Quoted in Peter Jaret, "The Disease Detectives," *National Geographic*, January 1991, p. 34.
7. Quoted in ScienceDirect, "Cohort Studies," 2021. www.sciencedirect.com.
8. Brenda Wilson, "AIDS Study Marks 25th Year," *All Things Considered*, NPR, April 24, 2009. www.npr.org.
9. Andrew W. Artenstein, "The Discovery of Viruses: Advancing Science and Medicine by Challenging Dogma," Science Direct, 2012. www.sciencedirect.com.

Chapter Two: The Mystery of Sleeping Sickness

10. Quoted in Dana L. Bivens, "African Sleeping Sickness in British Uganda and in Belgian Congo, 1900–1910: Ecology, Colonialism, and Tropical Medicine," VCU Scholars Compass, 2015. https://scholarscompass.vcu.edu.
11. Victoria Austin, "African Trypanosomes—Where Did They Go?," *BugBitten* (blog), BioMed Central, February 3, 2017. https://blogs.biomedcentral.com.

12. David Bruce, *Preliminary Report on the Tsetse Fly Disease, or Nagama, in Zululand*. Durban, South Africa: Bennett and Davis, 1895, p. 2.
13. W.J. Tulloch, "Sir David Bruce: A Tribute," *Journal of the Royal Army Medical Corps.*, April 1955, p. 86.
14. Tulloch, "Sir David Bruce," p. 90.

Chapter Three: The Mystery of Polio in the Blood

15. Quoted in David M. Oshinsky, *Polio: An American Story*. New York: Oxford University Press, 2005, p. 126.
16. Quoted in David M. Oshinsky, "Breaking the Back of Polio," Yale School of Medicine, 2005. https://medicine.yale.edu.
17. Quoted in Heather A. Carleton, "Putting Together the Pieces of Polio: How Dorothy Horstmann Helped Solve the Puzzle," *Yale Journal of Biological Medicine*, June 2011. www.ncbi.nlm.nih.gov.

Chapter Four: The Mystery of the Dead Legionnaires

18. Quoted in Christopher Klein, "Remembering the Legionnaires' Outbreak," History.com, 2020. www.history.com.
19. Quoted in Elana Gordon, "40 Years Later, Scientist Who First Discovered Legionnaires' Disease Is Still Learning Lessons," WHYY, July 28, 2016. https://whyy.org.
20. Quoted in Klein, "Remembering the Legionnaires' Outbreak."
21. Quoted in Gordon, "40 Years Later, Scientist Who First Discovered Legionnaires' Disease Is Still Learning Lessons."
22. David Burke, "The Haunting World of Disease Detectives," RealClear Science, November 14, 2013. www.realclearscience.com.

Chapter Five: The Mystery of HIV/AIDS

23. Quoted in Michael Helquist, "Pioneer Reported First AIDS Cases in 1981; I Interviewed Him on the 5th and 20th Anniversaries," Michael Helquist (website), June 5, 2016. www.michaelhelquist.com.
24. Quoted in Elizabeth Fee and Daniel M. Fox, eds., *AIDS: The Making of a Chronic Disease*. Berkeley: University of California Press, 1992, p. 58.
25. Helen Branswell, "HIV's Genetic Code, Extracted from a Nub of Tissue, Adds to Evidence of Virus' Emergence in Humans a Century Ago," Stat, July 16, 2019. www.statnews.com.

26. Patrick Tang et al., "Infection Control in the New Age of Genomic Epidemiology," *State of the Science Review*, February 1, 2017. www.ajicjournal.org.

Chapter Six: The Mystery of Deadly Ebola in Africa

27. Quoted in Australian Center for Health Security, "The 'Disease Detective' on Ebola's Case," 2019. https://indopacifichealthsecurity.dfat.gov.au.
28. Quoted in Australian Center for Health Security, "The 'Disease Detective' on Ebola's Case."
29. Tom Koch, "Ebola in West Africa: Lessons We May Have Learned," *International Journal of Epidemiology*, February 2016. https://academic.oup.com.
30. Peter Piot et al., "Emergent Threats: Lessons Learnt from Ebola," *International Health*, September 2019. https://academic.oup.com.

Chapter Seven: The Mystery of the Virus from Wuhan

31. Quoted in Tara McKelvey, "Coronaviruses: Disease Detectives Track an Invisible Culprit," BBC, July 6, 2020. www.bbc.com.
32. Editors of *Nature*, "How Epidemiology Has Shaped the COVID Pandemic," *Nature*, January 27, 2021. www.nature.com.
33. Editors of *Nature*, "How Epidemiology Has Shaped the COVID Pandemic."
34. Marc Lipsitch, "Good Science Is Good Science: We Need Specialists, Not Sects," *European Journal of Epidemiology*, June 20, 2020. https://link.springer.com.
35. Seema Yasmin, "Disease Detectives Investigate Outbreaks at Home and Abroad," *Scientific American*, 2014. https://blogs.scientificamerican.com.

ORGANIZATIONS AND WEBSITES

American College of Epidemiology (ACE)
www.acepidemiology.org

The ACE promotes the science of epidemiology as a crucial tool in fighting disease. The group sponsors scientific meetings and aids would-be epidemiologists by helping expand their educational opportunities. The website contains helpful COVID-19 resources, including links to articles in the *Journal of the American Medical Association* (*JAMA*).

American Public Health Association (APHA)
www.apha.org

APHA promotes better public health in the United States by bringing together and pooling knowledge among a wide range of medical and public health organizations and professionals, including epidemiologists. The website tells how to earn college credits for courses in medicine and health care and lists job openings in those areas.

Coronavirus Disease (COVID-19), US Department of Labor/OSHA
www.osha.gov/SLTC/covid-19

This excellent site contains numerous links leading to a wide range of information about COVID-19, including medical facts, symptoms, control and prevention, how workers can avoid contracting the virus, the importance of wearing masks, and much more.

International Epidemiological Association (IEA)
www.ieaweb.org

With more than one thousand members in more than one hundred nations, the IEA promotes regular communication and sharing of ideas and research among epidemiologists everywhere.

The website features a colorful map that tells "What's happening in your region," plus a collection of articles containing the most recent news about epidemiology around the world.

Pandemics That Changed History, History.com

www.history.com/topics/middle-ages/pandemics-timeline

This informative site presents an overview of many of history's largest disease outbreaks, including those caused by cholera, leprosy, measles, bubonic plague, and HIV/AIDS. The authors provide several links to other articles that cover related material.

FOR FURTHER RESEARCH

Books

Barbara Krasner, *Pandemics and Outbreaks*. New York: Greenhaven, 2020.

Joshua Loomis, *Epidemics: The Impact of Germs and Their Power*. Nashville: Turner, 2020.

Hal Marcovitz, *The COVID-19 Pandemic: The World Turned Upside Down*. San Diego: Brightpoint, 2020.

Harmindar K. Sran Rehs, *Washing Germs Down the Drain!!* Denver: Outskirts, 2020.

Sonia Shah, *Pandemic: Tracking Contagions, from Cholera to Coronaviruses and Beyond*. New York: Picador, 2020.

Internet Sources

Boston University School of Public Health, "John Snow—the Father of Epidemiology," 2015. https://sphweb.bumc.bu.edu.

Centers for Disease Control and Prevention, "COVID-19 Vaccine," 2021. www.cdc.gov.

College of Physicians of Philadelphia, "Ebola Virus Disease and Ebola Vaccines," 2018, https://ftp.historyofvaccines.org.

Johnny Denenea, "The History of Legionnaires' Disease," Legionnaires' Lawyer, 2021. https://thelegionnaireslawyer.com.

Steve Hendrix, "A Mystery Illness Killed a Boy in 1969; Years Later, Doctors Believed They'd Learned What It Was: AIDS," *Washington Post*, May 15, 2019. www.washingtonpost.com.

Owen Jarus, "20 of the Worst Epidemics and Pandemics in History," Live Science, March 20, 2020. www.livescience.com.

Andrew Joseph, "'A Huge Experiment': How the World Made So Much Progress on a COVID-19 Vaccine So Fast," Stat, July 30, 2020. www.statnews.com.

Christopher Klein, "Remembering the Legionnaires' Outbreak," History.com, 2020, www.history.com.

Public Health, "HIV and AIDS: An Origin Story," 2021. www.publichealth.org.

Public Health Online, "A Guide to Careers in Epidemiology," 2021. www.publichealthonline.org.

Tsetse.org, "David Bruce." www.tsetse.org.

Tulsa Heath Department, "Epidemiologists Are Disease Detectives." www.tulsa-health.org.

Seema Yasmin, "The CDC's 'Disease Detectives' Are Our Front-Line Defense Against Coronavirus," *Rolling Stone*, February 29, 2020. www.rollingstone.com.

INDEX

Note: Boldface page numbers indicate illustrations.

AIDS (acquired immunodeficiency syndrome), 13, 36–41
   discovery of organism causing, 40
   first known US case of, 39
American College of Epidemiology (ACE), 58
American Public Health Association (APHA), 58
Artenstein, Andrew W., 15
Austin, Victoria, 18–19

bacterium, definition of, 33
Bruce, David, 16–22
Burke, David, 35

Cantor, Eddie, 26
case control studies, 11–12
   on risk for contracting PCP, 37–38
case series (clinical) studies, 9
   on cataracts in babies, 10–11
   on COVID-19, 49
   definition of, 11
   on Ebola, 43–44
cholera
   1853 London epidemic, 4, 8
   birth of epidemiology and, 6–7
   death toll from, 5
   outbreak in Guinea-Bissau, 11–12
Christy, Cuthbert, 16–17
cohort studies, 12–13
   on HIV transmission, 39
contact tracing, definition of, 49
Coronavirus Disease (COVID-19), US Department of Labor/OSHA (website), 58
COVID-19, 48–54
   deaths from, 49
   impact of mask wearing on, 52
   investigation into source of, 50–52
   patients with, **53**

Daltry, Daniel, 48
Denenea, Johnny, 35

Ebola, 15, 42–47
   case series studies on, 43–44
   genetic studies on, 46–47
   investigation into spread of, 43–45
Eley, Susannah, 5
epidemiology
   birth of, 6–7
   development of methods in, 9–10
   genomic, 41

field studies, 9, **10**
   challenges of, 47
   definition of, 9
food-borne illnesses, hepatitis A, 12
Fulton, John F., 29

Gallo, Robert C., 40
Gandhi, Monica, 52
genes, definition of, 41
genetic studies
   in Ebola research, 47
   on HIV, 41
genomic epidemiology, definition of, 41
Gottlieb, Michael, 36
Gregg, Norman McAlister, 10–11

hepatitis A, 12
HIV (human immunodeficiency virus), 13, 36–41
   means of transmission discovered, 38–39
   search for origins of, 40–41
Horstmann, Dorothy M., 23–24, 25–29, **27**

influenza (flu), 14–15
International Epidemiological Association (IEA), 58–59

Johns Hopkins University Coronavirus Resource Center, 49

Koch, Tom, 44–45

Laake, Petter, 12–13
Legionella pneumophila, 34

Legionnaires' disease, 15, 30–35
   deaths from, 35
   identification of organism causing, 34
Lipsitch, Marc, 54
localized, definition of, 45

March of Dimes, 26, 28
Massachusetts Department of Public Health, 12
McDade, Joseph, 30, 31, 32, 33–34, **34**
microscopes, 8, **14**, 14–15
Multicenter AIDS Cohort Study (MACS), 13
mutation, definition of, 46

nagama, 18–19
   definition of, 18
Nature (journal), 52

Pandemics That Changed History, History.com (website), 59
patient zero, definition of, 54
Paul, John R., 26
Payne, Thomas, **32**
PCP. *See Pneumocystis carinii* pneumonia
Piot, Peter, 47
Pneumocystis carinii pneumonia (PCP), 36–37
   definition of, 37
polio/poliomyelitis, 15, 23–29
   animal experiments with, 28–29
   outbreaks of, 24
   paralytic, 24
   research on vaccine for, 28
   virus causing, **25**

propagate, definition of, 21

Rayford, Robert, 39
Roosevelt, Franklin D., 26
Roper, Katrina, 42–43
  on challenges of fieldwork, 47
rubella (German measles), 11

Sabin, Albert B., 28
Salk, Jonas, 28
Shaffer, Nathan, 11–12
Shelby, Tyler, 48, 49
sleeping sickness
  (trypanosomiasis), 16–22
  examination of patient with, **18**
  investigation into, 18–21
  prevalence of, 20
  role of tsetse fly in spread of, 21–22
  symptoms of, 16
Snow, John, 4–7, 8

social distancing, definition of, 51

Thelle, Dag S., 12–13
trypanosomiasis
  definition of, 17
  See also sleeping sickness
tsetse fly, **21**
Tulloch, W.J., 22

Uganda, 16

Victoria (queen of England), 4
virus(es)
  causing poliomyelitis, **25**
  definition of, 13
  discovery of, 15

Wilson, Brenda, 13
World Health Organization, 20
Worobey, Michael, 41

Yasmin, Seema, 54